# Critical acclaim for
## *The Carbohydrate Addict's Diet*

"UPBEAT, POSITIVE ADVICE FOR WEIGHT-LOSS SUCCESS!"
*—Library Journal*

"A move in the right direction . . . takes much of the onus for obesity—or simply being overweight—off the individuals who suffer." *—Kansas City Star*

"Weight loss without deprivation." *—American Bookseller*

"Provocative . . . The Hellers describe carbohydrate addiction and its solution . . . and cite 109 references to support their ideas." *—The Detroit News*

"These researchers believe they have identified a cure for obesity . . . and cite a biological origin for weight gain and outline a strategy to correct it." *—Columbus Dispatch*

"TWO OF AMERICA'S LEADING RESEARCH SCIENTISTS HAVE DISCOVERED A CURE FOR FOOD ADDICTS." *—Star*

---

**Richard F. Heller,** M.S. Ph.D., is a research and health biologist and professor in the Department of Pathology at New York's Mount Sinai School of Medicine as well as in the Department of Biomedical Sciences of the Graduate Center of the City University of New York (CUNY). He is also Professor Emeritus of Biology and Medical Laboratory Technology at CUNY. **Rachael F. Heller,** M.A., M.Ph., Ph.D., is a research and health psychologist and professor at Mount Sinai School of Medicine and the Department of Biomedical Sciences of the Graduate Center of CUNY. The Hellers are the authors of the bestselling *The Carbohydrate Addict's Diet, The Carbohydrate Addict's Gram Counter*, and *Healthy for Life*.

D0051428

# *The* CARBOHYDRATE ADDICT'S PROGRAM *for* SUCCESS

## Taking Control of Your Life and Your Weight

## Dr. Rachael F. Heller and Dr. Richard F. Heller

A PLUME BOOK

A NOTE TO THE READER
The ideas, procedures, and suggestions contained in this book are not intended as a substitute for psychological counseling or consultation with your physician. All matters regarding your health require medical supervision.

PLUME
Published by the Penguin Group
Penguin Putnam Inc., 375 Hudson Street,
New York, New York 10014, U.S.A.
Penguin Books Ltd, 27 Wrights Lane, London W8 5TZ, England
Penguin Books Australia Ltd, Ringwood, Victoria, Australia
Penguin Books Canada Ltd, 10 Alcorn Avenue,
Toronto, Ontario, Canada M4V 3B2
Penguin Books (N.Z.) Ltd, 182–190 Wairau Road, Auckland 10, New Zealand

Penguin Books Ltd, Registered Offices: Harmondsworth, Middlesex, England

First published by Plume, an imprint of Dutton NAL,
a member of Penguin Putnam Inc.

First Printing, March, 1993
16   15   14   13   12   11

REGISTERED TRADEMARK—MARCA REGISTRADA

LIBRARY OF CONGRESS CATALOGING-IN-PUBLICATION DATA:
Heller, Rachael F.
    The carbohydrate addict's program for success : taking control of your life and your weight / Rachael F. Heller and Richard F. Heller.
        p.   cm.
    ISBN 0-452-26933-4
    1. Low-carbohydrate diet.    I. Heller, Richard F. (Richard Ferdinand), 1936–
    II. Title.
    RM237.73.H454   1992
    613.2'8—dc20                                                                92-33597
                                                                                          CIP

Printed in the United States of America
Set in Garamond Light
Designed by Eve L. Kirch

BOOKS ARE AVAILABLE AT QUANTITY DISCOUNTS WHEN USED TO PROMOTE PRODUCTS OR SERVICES. FOR INFORMATION PLEASE WRITE TO PREMIUM MARKETING DIVISION, PENGUIN PUTNAM INC., 375 HUDSON STREET, NEW YORK, NEW YORK 10014.

To Dr. Lee Salk, whose advice, clear thinking, and enthusiasm
have helped us immeasurably

and

To the hundreds of thousands of carbohydrate
addicts with whom we have worked or
who have written to us—whose stories,
experiences, challenges, and triumphs
have helped to enrich this book, our work, and our lives.

# Acknowledgments

We wish to express our appreciation to the following people:

Alexia Dorszynski—our editor, whose guidance, wise counsel, and very hard work have helped to make this book a source of pride as well as a tool for change.

Deb Brody—our editor, whose attentive response to our needs and the needs of the project have insured its quality.

Lisa Johnson for her unswerving energy and in acknowledgment of her fine professional judgment and to her assistant, Tracey Guest, who has helped us when we needed it most and to the many other editors and staff at Penguin.

Elaine Koster and Arnold Dolin—our publishers, for their continued integrity and commitment.

Melissa Jacoby—Art Director, for her fine artistic talents.

Mel Berger of The William Morris Agency—the best agent known to man (or woman). His years of experience, well-thought-out advice, good common sense, creativity, patience, and very, very hard work have helped us every step of the way.

Professor Ronald E. Gordon, Ph.D., Director of Electron Microscopy, Department of Pathology, Mount Sinai School of Medicine, and Mr. Norman Katz, Supervising Technologist of Electron Microscopy, Department of Pathology, Mount Sinai School of Medicine, and his wife, Madeline—for their helpful suggestions, comments, and encouragement.

Professor Alan L. Schiller, M.D., Chairman, Department of Pathology, Mount Sinai School of Medicine—for his insights, enthusiasm, and support.

Sharon Althea Smith and Ana Luisa Vazquez, the finest of all research assistants, whose industriousness, intelligence, and commitment make our research possible and our lives most enjoyable.

The Apple Computer Company—for developing the powerful, user-friendly Powerbook 170 computers that were invaluable in the preparation of all written and graphic materials.

# Contents

## PART III.  YOUR MIND: YOUR WILL TO WIN

# Introduction

I am what I am.
                            —Popeye the Sailorman

As far as we know, Popeye is one of a rare breed—he accepts himself for what he is. Of course, he and Olive Oyl never were overweight, nor did they have the frustration, fear, pain, or self-blame that often goes along with it. For those of us who are, self-acceptance is not so easy. We are so busy blaming ourselves for our weight problems that we simply don't listen to what our bodies and our own experience are telling us. Instead of paying attention to what we already know about ourselves, we listen to the advice of friends and family who in turn get their information from advertisers whose sole job is to sell the latest in their "quick-fix" solutions. Though we wouldn't use a friend's eyeglasses or a sister-in-law's medication, we eagerly embrace their latest fad diet discovery in one more attempt to gain control of our eating and our weight.

---

**I don't understand *why* I lose control.
Why can't I do this one thing in my life?**

---

"I should be able to lose weight and keep it off. It's just a matter of willpower," we tell ourselves.

"But I get so hungry," a voice inside replies. "I don't understand

**1**

*why* I lose control. I do other things well. Why can't I do this one thing in my life?"

"Because you're not trying hard enough," we yell back. "Just use a little self-control. It won't kill you. Don't be such a baby."

Eventually, the voice that asks "why" is ashamed and speaks no more. If we bully ourselves long enough or loudly enough, we stop speaking up for ourselves. For the carbohydrate addict "why" questions are the most important questions of all. *Why* you get hungry, *why* you lose control, *why* you put weight on easily, *why* you blame yourself, and *why* you have failed in the past, are very, *very* important. They hold the answers to *how* to conquer the patterns of past and *how* to make a future that will bring you the joy and success you deserve.

## Your Own Special Journey

There is a prayer that says *"Grant me the serenity to accept the things I cannot change, the courage to change the things I can, and the wisdom to know the difference."* Most of us go from the accepting part of the prayer to the changing part of the prayer and back to the accepting part again without ever getting to the third part, the part about the wisdom. We try with all of our might to lose weight and to keep it off, to change what we *think* we should be able to change, to control our eating "once and for all." We tell ourselves that losing weight will put an end to the sadness, the deprivation, the frustration, and the injustices that we have endured.

Sometimes we are successful in losing weight, sometimes not. Sometimes we keep the weight off for a little while; sometimes we become dissatisfied and discouraged and we give up. We flip back and forth between trying to control our desire to eat and trying to accept the fact that sometimes we are being controlled by it. And even when we are successful in our weight loss, we come face-to-face with the reality that our cravings for carbohydrates result in a great deal more than just some extra pounds; the self-blame and shame that goes along with it can affect our mind, our body, and our feelings.

---

**The Carbohydrate Addict's Program for Success
is about *you* and your journey through life.**

---

*The Carbohydrate Addict's Program for Success: Taking Control
of Your Life and Your Weight* is about the third part, the wisdom
part, of the Serenity Prayer. It is about bringing an end to struggle,
denial, feelings of failure, frustration, sadness, anger, self-blame,
and pain so that you may be free to take control of your life and
your weight. It's about understanding the difference between what
*is,* what *should be,* and what *could be.* It's about making choices.
Most important, it is a book about *you* and your journey through
life.

# Traveling Light

As we travel through life, each of us accumulates baggage. This
baggage consists of broken promises, lost trust, betrayals, fears, and
unfair treatment. Baggage may come from our parents, from family
members, from friends, lovers, acquaintances, and even strangers.
The more baggage that we accumulate, the more burdensome and
difficult is our journey.

Many of us have stopped on the road of life, stuck because we
can barely move under the weight of our baggage. Some of us know
that we are stuck and are willing to face it, some of us don't even
want to acknowledge it. Some of us are stuck in relationships or
jobs that are filled with stress, ridiculously demanding, and ultimately thankless. We find ourselves striking out for no reason or,
worse, seething inside while we smile and politely swallow our anger. We may experience mood swings, feeling wonderfully exhila-
rated one minute, then sad or hopeless the next. We may find
ourselves tired and unmotivated, feeling "blah" for no reason that
we can understand.

---

**The pride that we feel in our weight loss is
followed by the crush of defeat when the lost
weight is regained.**

---

For carbohydrate addicts, life's baggage is doubly heavy because we also bear the blame from our families, friends, the world, and worst of all, ourselves, for the hunger, weight, and health problems that are associated with carbohydrate addiction. Even trusted friends may talk about us behind our backs. We blame ourselves for each diet slip-up, telling ourselves that all we need to do is "use a little willpower."

If we do succeed in losing weight, the pride that we feel in our weight loss is almost always followed by the crush of defeat when the lost weight is regained. The thoughtless comments or jokes of friends and strangers, the accusations from physicians who haven't taken the time and trouble to understand us, all add to the baggage we carry. Soon we find that we can no longer move.

Now is the time to let go of this baggage: the rules that don't work, the beliefs that have let you down, the discarded promises, the disappointing relationships, the fruitless hopes, and the unanswered prayers that keep you from finding and enjoying your own Circle of Success. It is time to discover the essential *you* that is the most vital component of your Circle of Success—and in doing so, to take control of your life and your weight.

---

**It is time to let go of the baggage that we all carry: the rules that don't work, the promises that let you down, the disappointing relationships. It is time to bring out the essential you.**

---

This book contains many exercises that will help you to replace the negative experiences of your past—your baggage—with current, positive, living triumphs. You will come to know the exhilaration of traveling light through your journey, no longer burdened with the rules, pain, and failure of the past.

The Experiences that we have included in *The Carbohydrate Addict's Program for Success* are the results of our own personal pain, our struggles, failures, and victories, as well as nine years of helping thousands of others with their challenges and victories. We have been where you stand now, and we will help you on your journey.

# Discovery and Recovery: The Path of the Past, Present, and Future

This book will guide you in the two most important tasks in life. The first task is to allow the thoughts and feelings that you have held inside for so many years to rise to the surface and be experienced. We call that task Discovery. The second task is to throw off the negative influences of these experiences and to replace them with positive thoughts and feelings that will help you to achieve the goals that *you* want for yourself. We call this second task Recovery. Together, Discovery and Recovery will lead you to complete your own Circle of Success.

## Your Own Personal Path

Discovery will take place as each Experience helps you to explore your past and your present. *Past* sections of the chapter will help you to reexperience, in vivid detail, the thoughts, feelings, and physical sensations that you have known and, perhaps, forgotten. *Present* sections will help to uncover the ideas, emotions, and feelings that you continue to carry from the past into your life today.

The *Future* section of each chapter will help you to know Recovery—the triumph of throwing off the pain, frustration, and self-blame, the deprivation, fear, and failure of the past. You will find yourself free to complete your Circle of Success without conflict or self-sabotage. You will come to know what is important to *you* and how best *you* can get it. As you complete both the Discovery and Recovery sections of each chapter, you will find that you are free to accept and enjoy what life has to offer.

It is vital that you balance Discovery and Recovery. Some people become mired in discovering and rediscovering their pasts. They tend to dwell on what "could" or "should" be and end up blaming others for their current problems. Unmotivated and unhappy, they are unable or unwilling to pull themselves out of their "rut." Other people, working alone or with professional guidance, try to jump too quickly into Recovery, without learning from the past or examining the present. They are likely to lose ground and fail when they come face-to-face with a real and immediate difficulty. When the challenge of Discovery and the triumph of Recovery are used together, however, you find yourself free to appreciate all that you are and to gather around you people who will truly value and appreciate you. The Discovery and Recovery that you achieve in working through the Past, Present, and Future sections of each Experience will help you to achieve and complete your own personal Circle of Success.

## Forgetting, Remembering, Understanding

There is an old Chinese proverb that says *"I hear and I forget. I see and I remember. I do and I understand."* Our own lives bear this out. Each of us has remembered and forgotten our own thoughts, ideas, and feelings a thousand times, rarely *doing* anything with them. Memories move like breezes (sometimes, more like hurricanes—through our minds) but no matter how strong they are, we pay them little more than passing attention. We usually allow them simply to pass away. Similarly our thoughts and feelings are fleeting. We seldom take the time to explore them, giving very little importance to them. Instead, we react for the moment and go about our business. But that well of unexplored thoughts and feelings is a great deal deeper than we think. Feelings buried inside of us influence every part of our daily lives: our relationships, our work, our opinions of ourselves and of others.

---

**The burden of unresolved pain that carbohydrate addicts carry is heavier than most. In a world that does not understand them and often blames them, carbohydrate addicts bear the scars and the shame of other people's ignorance.**

---

The burden of unresolved pain that carbohydrate addicts carry is heavier than most. In a world that does not understand us, in a world that blames us for what is a physical imbalance, a metabolic disorder, carbohydrate addicts bear the scars and the shame of other people's ignorance. Some of us have been able to lift the physical addiction, to stop the cravings and to remove the burden of the excess weight; others have not as yet broken free. But whether or not being overweight is still a factor, the burden of years of blame, frustration, deprivation, and self-doubt may still remain.

---

**Whether or not being overweight is still a concern of yours, the burden of years of blame, frustration, deprivation, and self-doubt may still remain.**

---

## What Lies Ahead

We do not think that it is enough for you to hear about our experiences or even about the experiences of others. It is *you,* and your experiences, that count. In the pages that follow, we will interact with you, and you with us. We will share our experiences and the experiences of others, but we will also help you explore your experiences, your hopes, your needs, along with your determination to succeed.

As with anything new, you may find that you feel uneasy or self-conscious as you begin the Experiences in this book. You may put them off for a while without knowing why. Or you may find them exciting and challenging from the start. The Experiences that follow are not terribly demanding or difficult, but they do require that you set aside time to do them and that you be willing to be open and honest with yourself. Remember: No one will be looking over your shoulder, nobody will be judging you or criticizing you. Your answers will not be evaluated or given a grade. They are your answers. They reflect that unique entity we call "you." There are no wrong answers, there are only your answers, and by definition, they are right.

If it seems hard to put aside time in what already looks like an impossible schedule, remember that this time is for you; you are building toward your own success. Imagine that a family member needed help for five or ten minutes a day. You would help them find the time, wouldn't you? If you were told that your dog's or your cat's health depended on your doing a chore that would take ten or fifteen minutes a day, you would find the time for that, wouldn't you? Well, let's just say, you have to be as important as any other family member and certainly as important as a dog or cat!

If you find that you are reluctant to begin the Experiences or reluctant to continue working on a particular one, if you put it off time after time, that in itself may be an important sign. Reluctance is often a signal that we are faced with a task that we would rather ignore or avoid because of pain or fear, that we don't want to face something or that we're concerned about failing at it. When reluctance rears its ugly little head, you must be prepared to "gently overcome." It is important for you to hold your head up high and forge ahead. You must make a commitment to taking the time to work through the book, to getting in touch with the pain, sadness, and anger, and in doing so, to let go. Often the stronger the resistance, the more you need to rid yourself of it. Trust in yourself: trust that you are strong enough to let it in, to let it out, and to let it go.* We have been there and we will be with you every step of the way.

Each set of Past and Present Discovery Experiences that you complete will represent a part of your life—along with the pain, disappointment, frustration, or deprivation that may have held you prisoner. As you complete each Past and Present Experience, you will be asked to destroy it. As you destroy Experience after Experience, the book will decrease in size, and your storehouse of pain, guilt, anger, deprivation, and shame will also decrease. This sets the path for your Recovery. Each Future Experience may be saved and reread over and over, and with it you will be free to enjoy your very own Circle of Success.

*This book is not meant as a substitute for psychotherapy. If you find that you are hesitant to deal with a particular area, or with feelings in general, you may wish to seek the individual help of a health professional in your area.

# A Hand of Friendship, a Noble Battle

This book offers us a chance to extend to you the hand of friendship, compassion, and understanding. We can talk with you, help you explore your thoughts, beliefs, and feelings, and offer you our personal guidance. We will interact with you, share with you our own experiences and the experiences of thousands and thousands of others who have written to us from around the United States, Canada, United Kingdom, Australia, Israel, South America, Germany, and New Zealand in response to our book, *The Carbohydrate Addict's Diet*.

In our nine years of research, we have found that 75 percent of people who are overweight, and many normal-weight folks as well, are carbohydrate-addicted. If you are not sure that you are carbohydrate-addicted, we recommend that you take the test in our book, *The Carbohydrate Addict's Diet*.

Please remember that you are the one person who knows more about *you* than anyone else in the world. Rather than listen to the so-called experts tell you that "one size fits all," that what is good for someone else is good for you, it is time to work alongside someone who can help *you* learn about *your* strengths and weaknesses, your skills, your patterns of thinking and reacting. Then and only then can you win your battle and put down the burden that you have been carrying.

---

**This is a noble battle, as noble as any battle for freedom. This is *your* battle for freedom.**

---

It is a noble battle, as noble as any battle for freedom. This is *your* battle for freedom. You are an army of one and as you have learned, no one can fight this battle for you. But remember, we will be there beside you, to guide you every step of the way.

Any soldier must be trained, must learn the lay of the land and the use of his weapons. You have the advantage of having lived in the territory, a major advantage in any battle. In your battle, avoid dwelling on the skirmishes that you have lost in the past. It will be far better now to concentrate on what you have learned from any of these defeats. The greater the number of your defeats, the more you will have learned. Each will provide a clue as to how better to fight the enemy in the future. You bring the key to your victory—your knowledge of yourself.

---

**The greater the number of your past defeats, the better! Each will furnish a clue as to how better to fight the enemy in the future. Past failures provide the key to your future victories.**

---

We will be beside you, guiding you through the Experiences that follow. We also bring the stories of many others who have fought and lost and fought again and finally won. The prayer for serenity, courage, and wisdom may end for the moment, but our lives go on and we are changed.

## As You Begin . . .

this book, we make the following suggestions:

1. Set aside a specific time or times each day and read a manageable section of this book and/or do a reasonable number of exercises. Remember, this time is for you and your needs.
2. Work at a pace that is comfortable for you. Do not try to complete more Experiences than you have time for. Rushing the job may get it done sooner, but will not result in a quality product at the end. By working slowly and consistently, you will reap the rewards of your work.
3. Each day, record your recollections, reflections, and thoughts about what you read and the exercises that you did the day before.
4. Don't try to be perfect. Do the best that you can for the moment and then let go. Perfectionism is a very hard taskmaster. Remember that your goal is to take care of yourself, not to blame or shame yourself into compliance.

As you progress through each of the Experiences that follow, you will begin to notice a change. Hesitation, concern, and reluctance will give way to excitement, pride, and a feeling of control—control over your body . . . and your life.

Let us begin the journey, now, together. We will be with you every step of the way.

# PART I

# The Emerging Circle

# CHAPTER 1

# Rachael and Richard: Roads Traveled

That which does not kill you, makes you strong.

—Proverb

## Rachael's Confession

For more than twenty years I lived a lie. I told everyone that the lie was true and everybody readily agreed that it was so. Most of the time I even believed it myself. But it was a lie and deep down inside I knew it.

The lie was that the things that I hated about my life were caused by being fat. "If I were thin . . ." I would say, and a list of ten lifetime dreams would come to mind.

---

**For more than twenty years I lived a lie.**

---

"If I were thin, I would leave that louse," I would tell myself. "If I were thin, I would buy all clothes that I want . . . and I'd look gorgeous . . . or I'd probably look great in just jeans and a T-shirt." "If I were thin, I'd pick the man I wanted, I'd pick out someone rich and famous, and I'd make a plan for meeting him. I'd pretend my car broke down in front of his house and . . ." "If I were thin, everything would be all right." My dreams knew no boundaries but one; they all started with "if I were thin. . . ."

My friends and family supported the lie. "If you were thin, you could have any guy you wanted," they would promise. "Men would beat down your door, if you were thin." I never wondered, if that was true, why there were so many slim women living alone, without the men of their dreams.

Even my doctors added their unfounded medical opinions to the "if you were thin" fantasy world. "If you lost weight, you wouldn't get backaches," they would assure me. "If you weren't so heavy, you wouldn't get sick so often."

I knew it was unreasonable to expect to live "happily ever after" based on weight alone, but everyone supported my things-to-come-if-you-were-thin world of illusion, and though I knew it wasn't the whole truth, I continued to blame all of my day-to-day problems on my weight. My friends and family alike allowed me to do it. As the years passed, my hopes and beliefs about a better life based on a slimmer body continued, and, indeed, grew stronger.

"If I were thin, I wouldn't take it anymore," I would tell myself. "I would say exactly what I thought. I wouldn't be afraid." "If I were thin, I would stop taking care of everyone else. Other people would take care of me, for once." "If I were thin, I wouldn't put up with his stuff anymore." "Oh, God. I could be so happy, if only . . . if only, I were thin."

---

**In a never-ending stream of broken promises, lost hopes, and wasted money, I submitted to every new eating plan or liquid fast that came down the pike.**

---

In a never-ending stream of broken promises, lost hopes, and wasted money, I submitted to diet regimen after diet regimen, taking on every new eating plan or liquid fast that came down the pike. I would lose weight for a time, but as you might suspect, my moments of victory did not last long. Up and down, up and down, I'd lose and regain, over and over again. Weight Watchers, Metrecal, Stillman's, Atkins, Weight Watchers again, Pritikin, the Rice Diet, the Grapefruit Diet, behavioral modification, hypnotism, fruit fasts, water fasts, liquid fasts. I tried them all. I'd suffer and give up the pleasure of eating the foods that I loved, and, in return, the pounds would slip away. But all the time I could feel the recurring cravings and the mounting hunger breathing down my neck. I lived in fear and in the knowledge that it was just a matter of time before I would give in and the weight would return. And, of course, it always did.

With each diet failure, I felt worse about myself. I would try to convince myself that all I had to do was "eat sensible meals." I would attempt to eat "reasonably." "Everything in moderation," I would caution myself—but my body knew nothing of moderation. Most sensible meals were followed, an hour or two later, by a "harmless snack" of fruit or "just one small bite of something sweet." Sooner or later, in a matter of days or in a matter of hours or in a matter of minutes, my eating would, once again, be out of control and anything in the house (or the nearby store) was up for grabs.

Because my attempts at losing weight and keeping it off always ended in failure, I could not understand that weight loss itself could never free me. No matter what anyone said, the only answer to my suffering that I could imagine was to lose weight. Only during brief moments of clarity did I catch glimpses of a larger picture with the fleeting insight that "perhaps weight alone is not my enemy."

I remember, many years ago, coming to this realization for the first time. I weighed well over 300 pounds at the moment and had just regained the 40 or so pounds that I had suffered to take off, along with an additional 12. I turned to my friend, Arleen, who was also quite overweight and I said, "You know, it's not the weight that's the problem. If somebody could make me thin tomorrow, it still wouldn't be any good if I were always fighting the hunger."

---

**"You know, it's not the weight that's the problem.
If somebody could make me thin tomorrow, it
still wouldn't be any good if I were always
fighting the hunger."**

---

My friend laughed in my face. "Oh, come on," she said. "If someone could make you thin tomorrow, are you telling me that you'd turn it down? Who are you kidding?" I felt ashamed and confused and figured that she was probably right and that I was just trying to make myself feel better. I never brought it up again and the insight pretty much disappeared from my mind.

Since then, I have come to understand that my addiction to carbohydrates was, is, and will always be my enemy. My addiction, and my addiction alone, robbed me of my dreams, my self-esteem, my self-control, and my dignity.

Today I am a size six (size 6!) and I have been for nine years. Now I know how right I was way back then for, as much as I love being thin, I would not be happy if I still lived in the throes and torment of my carbohydrate addiction. Being thin is wonderful but it, in itself, did not change my life. Losing my addiction and the pain and torment, the self-blame and shame that went along with that loss was much, much more important than the weight itself.

Today I am free to eat the foods I love in the quantities that satisfy me, every day. I am deprived of nothing. When I finish my meals, I feel complete. I don't worry about going off my program or worry about putting the weight back on. I enjoy my weight loss and my life. Today I feel good about myself; more than that, I do not judge myself or put myself on trial. I do not measure myself in fear of finding myself lacking. A true appreciation for my abilities and a forgiveness for any qualities that may be found lacking have replaced my tight, self-demanding nature.

---

**Happiness is not just being normal weight; it is feeling like a normal, healthy person.**

---

It is clear to us, and to the many carbohydrate addicts that we have helped, that happiness is not just being normal weight; it is feeling, sometimes for the first time in your life, like a normal, healthy person.

## Richard's Double Betrayal

The earliest memory that I have is that of sneaking back to the kitchen after dinner in order to get more dessert. After the meal, I had tried to wheedle more ice cream out of my parents, but my mother refused. I couldn't have been more than three years old, but I knew what the refrigerator was for and where the ice cream was kept. I wasn't able to reach the handle on the refrigerator, so I pulled over a chair and placed it squarely in front of the tightly closed door. Then I pulled and I pulled and I pulled. Whammo! I toppled to the floor.

My mother ran in to see her "chubby baby" covered with blood. Like magic she pushed aside the chair and easily reached into the promised land of the refrigerator that had eluded me a few moments before. As she reached in for some ice to stem the bleeding from my nose, I pointed to the ice cream and continued to wail. She pried open the container, handed me a spoon, and with her hand holding a handkerchief over my bloody nose, I finished my well-earned dessert. I have to admit, to that three-year-old it seemed like a pretty good trade-off.

---

**My brother was eight years older and referred to me as "the human garbage can." He delighted in stuffing me with food in front of his friends. They would all sit around and take bets as to when I might finally refuse to eat another mouthful of food.**

---

My brother was eight years older and referred to me as "the human garbage can." He delighted in stuffing me with food in front of his friends. They would all sit around and take bets as to when I might finally refuse to eat another mouthful of food. My brother figured he should be able to win more often because he had the inside dope on what I had eaten in the last day or so, but he never seemed to be the consistent winner. He later confessed that, contrary to what he would have expected, the more I ate, the more I could be counted on to consume still more. Now we understand that this is the trademark of the carbohydrate addict and one of the first signs of the physical disorder that lies within: the more I ate, the more I wanted.

---

**The more I ate, the more I wanted.**

---

It seemed as if I was always hungry. As a pudgy redheaded kid, I grew in both directions at the same time, and, for a while, my spurts in height compensated for my insatiable appetite. I had nearly reached my 6'2" adult height by the time I was sixteen. Suddenly, it seemed as if my body had betrayed me. The food that I had been able to enjoy until that time now turned quickly and easily into fat. I had to choose: temporary satisfaction followed by self-blame and shame, or self-righteous victory and maddening hunger. One side would win, then the other. From that time on I lived with a daily battle of will against my body's drive to eat.

---

**The food that I had been able to enjoy until that time now turned quickly and easily into fat.**

---

I was a handsome young man, intelligent and sensitive, but I knew that the "love handles" that hung over my waist made me less appealing to the girls. I wore large sweaters when they weren't in fashion. I wore open jackets in the summer, but I perspired profusely and looked like an old man afraid of catching a cold. When I convinced myself that these devices couldn't hide the way I looked, I decided to lose weight. Girls, I told myself, were more important than food. Now I understand that way of thinking is like saying that water is more important to survival than air. I wanted, and needed, both.

Committed to the fight for the female, I took on diet after diet, losing weight only to gain it back. Metrecal, a liquid diet program, then calorie counting gave way to skipping meals and semi-starvation. "I'm not hungry," I would tell my mother. She'd look at me as if I had said I was going to Mars for the afternoon, for she knew me better than that. Inevitably, the weight would come off. Then my hunger and cravings would override my resolve and soon I'd gain it all back again, plus a few extra pounds to spare.

When commercial programs and traditional diets failed, I invented some diets of my own. From somewhere I got the idea that lemon juice would burn off the excess fat. Rather than admit that I was trying to lose weight, I attempted to convince my friends and family that plain lemon water really was "very refreshing" and that "after all, citrus is supposed to be quite good for you." No one believed me, but no one was able to figure out what it was that I was trying to do.

My battle with my weight continued into my twenties. Each fall, the demands of working while going to school translated into the accumulation of additional pounds. Friends and family learned to expect to see me, like a squirrel, gathering my winter layer of fat as the days grew colder.

---

**Committed to the fight for the female, I took on diet after diet only to lose weight and then gain it back. The weight would come off, but my hunger and cravings would override my resolve. Soon I'd gain it all back again, with a few extra pounds to spare.**

---

By this time I had several different sets of clothes to accommodate my up-and-down weight changes and when I met the woman who was to become my wife, she commented on being impressed by my varied wardrobe. Little did she realize that each 15-pound increment meant a new set of formally abandoned garments.

Though she met me when I was at my high weight, my then-fiancée told me she loved me just the way I was. I was in heaven. I was loved though I was fat; I could still be accepted. What man could ask for more?

We married and though I secretly feared that her acceptance would allow me to become increasingly heavy, this was not the case. As the demands of our growing family increased, I worked full-time as a professor and, in addition, taught part-time at four different jobs. I managed to juggle an impossible schedule so that I was able to take care of the children, enabling my wife to return to school. I was as active as I had been as a very young man, and though I ate like two truck drivers, my weight held steady . . . for a time.

As I approached my late thirties, my body betrayed me once again. Though I was working just as hard and eating no more, pound by pound my weight increased. At first I attributed the extra inches to holiday celebrations, to a well-deserved vacation, or to grabbing too much food on the run. But soon it became an undeniable fact: my weight was clearly out of control.

My sense of betrayal was great. It didn't seem fair. I was eating no more, I was working from morning until night, and I was putting on pounds. I felt as if some bargain had been broken. I was keeping up my end but my body was reneging on the deal.

Even greater than my present concerns was my fear for the future. I was in my late thirties now. What would happen in my forties? Or fifties? Or sixties? I pictured myself like some flabby Dorian Gray, growing older and fatter rather than older and wiser. I tried to promise myself that I would just have to try harder to eat less but I knew that I was fooling myself; I had tried to eat sensibly in the past, and while I always lost weight, I always gained it back.

The next ten years of yo-yo dieting led me to discover that I had a physical problem that was driving me to eat and setting my body up to gain weight. My scientific background led me to investigate and discover the cause and the solution for this relatively common and simple physical malfunction.

Today I live with this understanding and the knowledge of how to control and correct the cause of my addiction. But what truly frees me is that the feelings of betrayal and self-blame of the past have been replaced by the joy and freedom of the present . . . and the miraculous promise of the future.

---

**The feelings of betrayal and self-blame of the past have been replaced by the joy and freedom of the present . . . and the miraculous promise of the future.**

---

## Happiness Fulfilled: A Personal Note to Our Readers

In our personal lives, as well as in our teaching and research at Mt. Sinai School of Medicine in New York and as directors of the Carbohydrate Addict's Center at Mt. Sinai Medical Center, through communications with the many people with whom we have worked personally and with the hundreds of thousands of readers who have bought and used *The Carbohydrate Addict's Diet* book, we have confirmed, over and over again, our early understanding: that excess weight is only one of the many barriers that may stand in the way of happiness.

Each of us is a great deal more than just our weight and so it is not surprising to find that even when the excess weight is lost, or when the addiction is no longer active, happiness still eludes us.

When you are unhappy, it is natural to assume that if you could just get rid of what makes you unhappy you would be fine. But it's not quite that simple.

---

**Happiness is more than the absence of unhappiness. You are not automatically happy merely because, at the moment, there is nothing making you unhappy.**

---

We have all had the experience of wondering why we were unhappy when "there's nothing to be unhappy about." But happiness is more than the absence of unhappiness. Happiness calls for an integration of mind and body and feelings. You do not feel automatically happy merely because, at the moment, there is nothing making you unhappy.

Each of us carries with us our past experiences and the feelings that are associated with them. True success then, must include the letting go of the negative experiences of the past and a healing of the mind, body, and feelings, so that we can experience the joy that is available to us now.

Being slim does not insure happiness, and, conversely, you need not be slim in order to be happy. A mind that is burdened with self-doubt and blame and with feelings that remain injured or scarred, will not be happy. Or free.

---

**This book is about freedom: freedom from pain, freedom from confusion and doubt, freedom from feeling like your life is not all that it can be.**

---

This book is about freedom: freedom from pain, freedom from confusion and doubt, freedom from feelings of failure, fear, shame or self-blame, freedom from feeling that perhaps your life is not all that it can be.

The pages that follow come from the lessons learned through pain, struggle, failure, and triumph—our own as well as others we have touched. It is the result of giving in, giving up, giving out, and trying one more time, and then, finally, succeeding. We share with you the rebirth that comes from discovering what few have ever known before and then seeing others benefit and fly free with the discovery.

You are about to embark on a wonderful journey. Though we have gone before you and will help you at every step along the way, this is your journey. Each discovery will bring you to another discovery until, without effort, you too find yourself free.

---

**You are about to embark on a wonderful journey.**
**Though we have gone before you and will**
**help you at every step along the way,**
**this is your journey.**
**Each discovery will bring you to another**
**discovery until, without effort, you too find**
**yourself free.**

---

# CHAPTER 2

# Carbohydrate Addiction:
# When the Victim Is Blamed

## What Is Carbohydrate Addiction?

**Car·bo·hy·drate Ad·dic·tion***  A compelling or recurring hunger, craving, or desire for carbohydrate-rich foods such as starches (bagels, bread, pasta, rice, and potatoes), snack foods (such as pretzels, popcorn, or potato chips), or sweets (including fruit and fruit juices, puddings, pies, cakes, ice cream, and chocolate).

Carbohydrate addicts often, although not always, have a tendency to easily gain weight; if some weight is lost through dieting, they have a tendency to easily regain the lost weight.

---

**When most carbohydrate addicts eat a full,
"healthy" breakfast, they find that they are
hungry before it's time for lunch.**

---

While a nonaddicted person can enjoy carbohydrates and feel satisfied, once carbohydrate addicts have a "taste" of the food they love, they have a very hard time stopping.

*See *The Carbohydrate Addict's Diet,* for a seventeen-item quiz that will help you determine if you are a mild, moderate, or severe carbohydrate addict and guide you in correcting the physical cause of your addiction.

Carbohydrate addicts are often stimulated to eat by the sight, smell, even the thought of food.

Some carbohydrate addicts feel "driven" to eat, even though, at times, they don't actually feel hungry.

Many carbohydrate addicts report that they are hungrier after a full breakfast than they would be if they had only had time for a cup of coffee (or nothing at all).

Carbohydrate addicts often find that they get tired and/or hungry in the middle of the afternoon.

Carbohydrate addicts often tell us that bread or pasta or sweets are their "diet downfall."

## The Telltale Signs

*Rachael and Richard:*

We both had all the signs that we now know are "telltale" of carbohydrate addiction but, at the time, no one seemed to recognize that there was such a disorder. We gained weight easily, eating not much more and, at times, perhaps less, than many of the other people we knew. Certainly, we would sometimes "indulge" and eat fattening foods but not enough to account for the weight that we seemed to put on so easily.

Once the weight was on, we found it very difficult to take off, especially as we passed forty. When we did succeed in losing weight, the extra pounds always crept (or sometimes leaped) back on. It was as if our bodies were fighting us—and, in fact, we now understand that they were.

---

**Carbohydrate addiction affects about 75 percent
of people who are overweight and many
normal-weight individuals as well. It usually
goes unrecognized, undiagnosed and,
of course, untreated.**

---

We now know that carbohydrate addiction affects about 75 percent of people who are overweight and many normal-weight individuals as well. The tragedy is that, in almost all cases, carbohydrate addiction goes unrecognized, undiagnosed, and, of course, untreated. Most physicians have little or no training in nutrition, eating, or weight problems, and most carbohydrate addicts are blamed by others and, of course, blame themselves.

---

**Carbohydrate addicts may be able to control their cravings for a while, but sooner or later, usually without warning, they lose control.**

---

Carbohydrate addicts may be able to control their cravings for carbohydrate-rich foods for a while, but sooner or later they find that they lose control, usually without warning. They may blame themselves or, in some cases, others around them, but the loss of control that they experience actually occurs when the body's insulin level is out of balance. The brain gets the message that there is a need to take in more food. The endocrine system gets the message that it should store the food that you take in as fat. If you find that sometimes you seem to "go blank" when you overeat or that you eat carbohydrate-rich food when you had no intention of "giving in," you may be experiencing nothing more than your body's overrelease of insulin. It is important that you understand that it may have nothing to do with willpower or strength.

## Not a Matter of Willpower, a Matter of Biology

Carbohydrate addicts are not weak-willed, they *do not* have a problem with willpower, even though they may have been taught to take the blame for what looks like a lack of control.

Psychological problems do not necessarily lie at the root of their eating either, but because carbohydrate addicts suffer the pain of struggling with their weight and the self-blame that comes with periodic loss of control, they may be left with the emotional scars that result from thinking that their eating and/or weight problems are their "fault." Scientific studies have *not* been able to find any consistent psychological trait or psychological problem that causes someone to overeat. That's because there is none. In fact, it is a wonder that more carbohydrate addicts do not have severe psychological problems—not as a cause of their eating but as a result of society's unfair treatment of them.

Many carbohydrate addicts have difficulty maintaining ideal weight. Because of the production of an excess of insulin (of which they are unaware), they will "naturally" have a tendency to gain weight, to keep the weight on, and, if they do lose it, to put it right back on.

Some of the carbohydrate addicts that we have seen at the Carbohydrate Addict's Center at Mt. Sinai Medical Center have weight problems that began early in childhood, but an equal number of carbohydrate addicts were normal weight when they were young and gained weight only as adults. Addiction triggers such as premenstrual changes, pregnancy, smoking cessation, lifestyle change, stress, or the simple act of getting older result in "adult onset" weight gain. If you gained weight as a result of this triggering, you probably feel somewhat betrayed. Once you were able to eat virtually what you wanted, or maybe you just had to keep an eye on your eating, then suddenly the whole thing got out of control. Here too, insulin is the key to the cause and the correction of the problem.

## Why Other Programs Have Failed You

In trying to gain control of their eating and their weight, carbohydrate addicts often turn to commercial programs or diets, but most of these programs fail because they do not treat the *cause* of the addiction. You may succeed at first, but failure is almost inevitable. Most commercial programs simply don't supply the carbohydrate addict's body with the nourishment it requires, in the way it needs it.

---

**Most commercial programs fail because they don't treat the *cause* of the addiction. You may succeed at first, but failure is almost inevitable.**

---

You may think that three "sensible" meals each day (with a snack) "should" be a good way to eat, but your body simply doesn't respond in the way that others do. When you try to feed it "sensibly," it keeps getting hungry. For the nonaddicted person, with normal insulin responses, three "sensible" meals a day, each containing small amounts of bread, fruit, or other carbohydrate-rich foods, is ideal; but for the carbohydrate addict, this regimen will make insulin levels spike and will result in carbohydrate cravings and weight gain. You may be okay for a while, but sooner or later your addiction will rear its head and the cravings and cheating will return. It has happened in the past and it will happen again in the future. Your body doesn't respond like other people's bodies. It's not a matter of willpower; it's a matter of biology.

Like almost all other carbohydrate addicts we, ourselves, tried the traditional diets (as well as many fads) over and over again. The commercial programs told us to eat "sensible" meals and although, at the start, we would manage to do it, in the end we would find ourselves out of control. The truth was that if we could manage to eat sensible meals, we wouldn't have had the weight problem in the first place.

Carbohydrate addiction has an effect on the mind *and* the body and, of course, on our feelings. When you do not understand the *cause* of your hunger or of your cravings, when you don't understand the cause of your struggle with control over food, your family, friends, co-workers, neighbors, even the reporters in the newspapers and on TV may convince you that you are being "indulgent" or even "self-destructive." If you fail to understand that a hormonal imbalance is causing the cravings and your loss of control, you may wrongly accuse and condemn yourself.

---

**If you fail to understand that a hormonal imbalance is causing the cravings and your loss of control, you may wrongly accuse and condemn yourself.**

---

When the two of us see someone struggling with their carbohydrate addiction, we know that our task is twofold. First, we help to restore the body's insulin balance and in doing so cut the cravings and weight gain. But restoring someone's physical balance is not enough. Our second task is to restore the psychological and emotional balance that is lacking after years of feelings of failure and self-blame.

The effect of carbohydrate addiction on feelings, on emotions, and on the spirit is enormous. Feelings of pride give way to shame; normal desires are open to self-ridicule. Because of misinformed so-called experts, carbohydrate addicts may come to doubt their very psychological health, wondering if fear of sex, fear of success, or tendencies toward self-destruction lie at the base of their eating problems. Because they are unaware that a physical imbalance is causing their bodies to crave carbohydrate-rich foods, many carbohydrate addicts experience a deep loss of self-esteem, mood swings, and may, at times, feel a sense of hopelessness. We help them to restore their bodies to a balance that they may never have before known and to find freedom and happiness that had, in the past, seemed like unreachable fantasies.

## The So-Called Diet Experts

*Rachael's Story:*

By the time I was in my teens, I had been to several "diet doctors." Somewhere along the way, I had heard that most physicians had no training in the area of eating or weight problems and very little training, if any, in nutrition. Still, it never, ever occurred to me to question their professional competence. One doctor, I remember, seemed to particularly enjoy embarrassing and shaming me. Each week he'd lean back in his big maroon leather office chair and begin: "You'll never be normal weight. *You* make the choices and it is only right that *you* suffer the consequences." He smiled as if he had the corner on truth and righteousness.

"Every time you reach into the refrigerator, you're telling the world that you *deserve* every extra pound that you carry. You look like a pig because you eat like one. There is nothing I nor anyone else can do for you." He smiled as he concluded his weekly summary of my fate and moved on to other business. He'd turn to folders on his desk or tell his secretary to place a phone call for him regarding another patient. He would dismiss me without the respect of a good-bye. He never gave me a chance to respond.

Even if he had given me an opportunity to tell him what I felt and what I experienced, I wouldn't have been able to make him understand. At the time, I could not explain *why* I ate the foods I did. I just found myself doing it. Sometimes I felt as if I barely knew what I was doing. It almost seemed that I had no ability to learn from one overeating episode to another. Often, I felt as if I were in a fog. I knew that I hated being fat and no matter what that doctor or anyone else said, I knew that I was not eating because I wanted to be fat. But I just couldn't seem to stop.

Each week, I would return to his office for more abuse and dutifully pay him the money my parents had given me for the visit. Then I would return home to report on my progress and submit to my parents' blame and frustration. I was coming to him for help and he was taking my money and enjoying his self-righteous abuse. How I would love to see him now!

It is sad but true that this kind of doctor didn't cease to exist twenty years ago. Any licensed physician can say he or she "specializes" in nutrition or dieting, although they have little or no specific training. Any nutritionist or dietician can say that they treat weight problems or eating problems, even though they use methods that fail 95 to 98 percent of the time. There is very little scientific evidence to back the diets that most experts recommend, and when we the dieter fails, they blame us and we blame ourselves as well!!

## The High Cost of Carbohydrate Addiction

If you're a carbohydrate addict, you have a hormonal imbalance (called *hyperinsulinemia*) that leads you to crave starches, snack foods, or sweets. This extra release of insulin takes place after you eat carbohydrates (starches, snack foods, fruits, or sweets) of any kind. The good news is that we know what causes this physical problem and we now know how to eliminate the cravings and remove the weight gain that goes along with it.

---

**You have probably been blaming yourself for a
condition that is simply *not your fault*.
We live in a world that blames us, the victims,
for a biologically based *physical* condition.**

---

Even though it is caused by a physical imbalance, carbohydrate addicts often blame themselves, or accept the blame of others, for a condition that is simply not their fault. If you think that you are a carbohydrate addict, you may have, at times, felt angry, isolated, frustrated, even hopeless when it comes to your eating or your weight. These feelings do not *cause* carbohydrate addiction but, rather, are the *result* of living in a world that is blaming you, the victim, for a physical condition that is simply *not your fault*.

We understand why you have these feelings and we know how to help you as well. The time for self-blame or accepting the blame of others for what is a hormonal imbalance is past. And that is what *The Carbohydrate Addict's Program for Success* is all about.

# CHAPTER 3

# Desperately Seeking Success

Self-trust is the first secret of success.
—Emerson

## Rachael's Broken Dream

After I lost 165 pounds, I expected my life to change. I waited for something to happen: for people to cheer, for fireworks to go off, for exciting men to beat a path to my door, for something to be different—radically different. But nothing happened. Oh, there were some people who congratulated me or told me how good I looked but, for the most part, except for my clothing size, nothing really changed. When people asked me how it felt to be slim for the first time in my life, I smiled and said "Terrific!" but my voice was a little too loud and a little too strained to be convincing.

Though I looked like a success, deep down inside I still felt like a failure. All my life I had dreamed of the moment when I would be thin and now it looked like it was going to be the biggest letdown of them all. What was worse, I had no other dream to depend on. I wanted my life to be different, I wanted to feel different, finally, finally, I wanted to feel like a success but the truth was, I didn't.

> **All my life I had dreamed of the moment when I would be thin. Now it looked like it was going to be the biggest letdown of them all.**

I was still in graduate school at the time, and I had been working with several people who had seen my weight loss and asked me to help them. It was a particularly low day for me, and as I sat across from one of my "success stories," Lana D., she told me that she wanted to lose more weight. Her doctor had said she was at a "good" weight and I asked her why she was pushing to lose more. She confided that she had always thought that losing weight would make her happy. Now that she had lost the weight, she still wasn't happy, and "Well," she confessed, "I guess I really don't know what else to do."

She continued, talking about her expectations and her disappointment. It was like looking into a mirror except that I was able to see in Lana what I had not seen in myself. For many years she had assumed that weight loss would lead to happiness. Now it was becoming clear that the one did not automatically follow the other. I began to understand and to help Lana see that *happiness did not automatically come from losing weight and losing weight did not automatically mean that you would be happy.* You could be a success at weight loss and still be unhappy. It happens every day. It happened to Lana and . . . it happened to me!

---

**For many years, Lana had assumed that weight loss would lead to happiness. Now it was becoming clear that the one did not automatically follow the other.**

---

## The Illusion of Success

I felt as if I had found the missing piece to a jigsaw puzzle. I had always assumed that if I were thin, I would be happy. I had always placed the blame for the unhappiness in my life on my failure to control my eating and my inability to control my weight. I had always said that if I was successful at that, nothing would stand in the way of my having a wonderful life. But now I had proved myself wrong. I was successful, but still I was not happy. So what was success? Certainly it involved achieving some goal that you set out for but, in addition, that goal had to make you happy. It couldn't just *promise* happiness, it had to deliver. I was beginning to see that success meant different things to different people.

For the guy I was dating (if you call it that), success meant the fulfillment of his ever-increasing desire to accumulate more and more things. It didn't really matter what he collected; he just seemed to need to own things, the more the better—comic books, videotapes, records, even people. Owning things made him happy. I guess one could say that in his own way he was a success. But you could see his desperation, his fear of not getting everything that he wanted. And from that point of view, he was a dismal failure.

For Lana, success meant looking good, but not just good—perfect. She told me that she would not be happy until her arms and tummy were tight "as a drum," and not a ripple could be seen as she stood naked in front of the mirror. She hated the stretch marks that her ample bosom had created and would not consider her weight loss successful until she could find someone who could remove the stretch marks and give her a "perfect body." Lana's happiness was based on an unattainable reality, and because of it, she was bound to be unsuccessful.

I knew that I, too, had to come to grips with what success meant for me and, as I was beginning to understand, that meant figuring out what made me happy and how to achieve it. I was in uncharted territory. Nobody I knew was really asking themselves what made them happy; most just seemed to kind of go on with their lives. A lot of my friends thought they were shooting for success by aiming for financial security. They assumed that lots of money would lead to lots of happiness. But that was because they had been living with money worries for so long. A few of my friends, now in their thirties, held a secret belief that finding the man of their dreams would make them happy. But that was because they had been living alone for so many years. As I looked around me, I saw the pattern. Each of us based our life's goals on the assumption removing the thing that made you unhappy would make you happy. But Lana and I knew that didn't work. There was more to happiness than getting away from what made you unhappy, but, at the time, I still didn't know what.

I wanted to talk to people about how they felt about their own lives, but I knew that it was just not something you bring up in conversation. It makes people uncomfortable to say the least. I could just imagine the interaction. "So tell me, so-and-so. Why do you think, after working so hard all of these years, you're still miserable?" No, that wasn't going to work.

---

**He laughed under his breath and mumbled something about my not knowing when I had it good. "I don't know what your problem is," he said, looking down at me disdainfully. "Maybe you just don't want to be happy. And maybe you pick friends who are as miserable as you are."**

---

At the time, I was "involved" with someone who loved to belittle me at every opportunity. When I tried to broach the subject, he laughed under his breath and mumbled something about the fact that maybe I just didn't know when I had it good. When I held my ground, saying that I really wasn't happy and that many of the people I saw around me weren't either, he came in for the attack. "I don't know what your problem is," he said, looking down at me disdainfully. "Maybe you just don't want to be happy. And maybe you pick friends who are as miserable as you are."

I asked for help and got a kick in the teeth. It's hard to look back now and imagine that I took it, but it was the kind of accusation I had heard all of my life. People used to say, "Maybe you just don't *want* to be thin." Now he was saying, "Maybe you just don't *want* to be happy."

But I *did* want to be thin and I *did* want to be happy. And something, something like the carbohydrates that had kept me heavy for so many years, something that I still didn't understand, remained in my life and was making me miserable.

I argued in my head for a week, defending myself in imaginary conversations, explaining my point of view. Finally, I stopped explaining and defending myself and threw off his accusations and then my own self-doubt, and I was on the trail again. I had a purpose. I told myself that I would track down the culprit that seemed to creep into my thinking and make me unhappy and, like the frequent carbohydrates that had kept me prisoner so long, I would eliminate it. I didn't understand exactly what I was doing, but I had a purpose and, ironically, I was happy in my pursuit.

> **I do my best work when someone tells me it can't
> be done. First I get scared and I start to wonder if
> I can do it. Then I become determined to show
> them that they are wrong.**

I do my best work when someone tells me it can't be done. First I get scared and I start to wonder if I can do it. Then I become determined to show them that they are wrong. Here, then, was my new challenge: to figure out why I was not happy. It didn't seem like a very noble cause; not one that you would brag about. It seemed rather self-centered, in fact. But I reasoned that if I had so much trouble achieving happiness, there were probably others who felt the same and, in time, I could share my discoveries with them. I no longer had the time to respond to my own feelings of unhappiness. I had a mission. "After all," I told myself, "feelings of unhappiness now are nothing more than symptoms to observe and learn about."

The scientist in me took over. I kept watch over my unhappiness in the same way that people with pain will mentally note its comings and goings in order to avoid it or to get the better of it. I took notes, mental and actual. I formulated guesses as to the cause of my feelings of sadness or fear or loneliness. I examined my own mood swings and moments of general discontent. Were they related to other people? Or what I ate? To certain situations? Or the level of my bank account? To my social life? My menstrual cycle? But with all the observing, noting, and thinking, nothing came together.

> **I could be poor but feel happy or just get a
> windfall of money and be miserable. I could be
> all alone and still be content or I could find
> myself going out with an attentive and handsome
> guy and still be worried and insecure inside. I
> couldn't figure it out.**

The only conclusion that I came up with was that my lack of joy, even in the face of my new svelte figure, took over at any time, in the company of anybody and was unrelated to money, my love life, or the time of the month. I noted that I could be poor but feel happy or just get a windfall of money and be miserable. I could be all alone and still be content or I could find myself out with an attentive and handsome guy and still be worried and insecure inside. I couldn't figure it out.

## The Revelation

*Rachael Continues:*

A few months later, at the time that I first met Richard, I felt stuck and unhappy. In our first conversation we discovered that we shared a lifetime of experiences. We were both carbohydrate addicts, we both had lost weight and had no trouble keeping it off. We were both very, very grateful to feel the driving need for food lifted but—and here was the catch—Richard was content. His wife of sixteen years had left him and, because of it, his relationship with his kids was suffering, he had grave financial concerns, but he was *happy*. Happy!

"Okay," I said to myself. "Either this guy is a fake or he's too dumb to know when he should be miserable." But Richard was neither and, even then, I sensed it. Deep down I wondered if, perhaps, he knew something I didn't know.

What followed had to be the craziest courtship in the world. I told Richard that I had a problem. I wasn't happy, I confided. I *should* be happy, and I thought I would be happy but I wasn't and I couldn't figure out why. He didn't think that I was strange (this I took as the mark of a very brave man). Instead, he complimented me on my honesty, saying that he thought I was terrific and that most people would never even challenge their own feelings. Then he offered to help me out. Maybe another perspective would be helpful, he said. Would I like him to try and help me figure out what was going on? "Would I ever," I thought. "Who could ask for more?"

"Maybe it's not *in* you to be happy," a voice inside whispered, but I knew it was the same voice that had told me that it wasn't "in me" to be thin. I had proved it wrong once and I would prove it wrong again. It was my old boyfriend's voice and I refused to listen to it. I knew that I wanted to be happy. Maybe Richard could help me figure out how.

---

**I still didn't understand exactly how he could help me if I didn't know what I needed. "That's my problem," Richard told me lovingly. "Let me help you figure that out."**

---

I still didn't understand exactly how he could help me if I didn't know what I needed. "That's my problem," Richard told me lovingly. "Let me help you figure that out." I'd been waiting all my life for Prince Charming to come and here he was. I wasn't going to let this one slip through my fingers. I told the voices inside my head that I had nothing to lose in trying and agreed that we'd work on it together.

First, Richard wanted to know what I had been doing in trying to deal with the problem myself. I told him that, when I found myself discontented, either sad, angry, or just plain blue, I would try to figure out what was going on inside me. But, I confessed, no pattern was coming through. He suggested that we attack it from the opposite angle. "Let's look at when you *are* happy. Let's see what's happening then. Let's look for a pattern at those times." It seemed logical and I had nothing to lose, just lots of attention from this delicious-looking guy. Still, it felt strange, like I shouldn't be doing it. But he seemed excited at the challenge, so I kind of went along for the ride.

At first, I couldn't see any "pattern," as he called it, in what made me happy. On one particular day, I noticed that I felt really good after I had done a favor for an old friend for whom I had a great deal of affection. I would have expected that. What I didn't understand was why, a few days later, I also felt good when I told someone at work exactly what I thought (which, to say the least, was not very complimentary). Two different behaviors, one nice and one apparently nasty, and both made me happy.

Later that week, I got a good mark on a paper I had written. I had worked very hard on the essay and I felt great when my grade reflected it. Nothing unusual in that. But when I got the same grade on a paper for a different course, for an essay I had thrown together the night before, I felt lousy. It didn't make sense. In both instances I received the same grade, but in one case I felt great and in the other, I felt terrible.

Neither the kind of deed nor the mark at school were the critical elements in my happiness. Two opposite kinds of deeds, one nice, one sort of nasty, and both led to feeling happy. Two good grades led to feeling happy in one case and feeling lousy in another. I told Richard that I thought that his "pattern" of happiness theory was going to prove a dead-end street.

Richard listened to my report and my conclusions. "Well, I wouldn't give up quite that fast," he said. "I think I have it." I wasn't impressed. What could he see that I didn't? Certainly, I knew myself better than he did after only a few weeks' time. "It has to do with your being in conflict; when different parts of you are in conflict, you can't be happy," he said. I pretended to be interested, but a part of me had stopped listening. "Don't you see," he continued, "a person isn't happy unless *all* of them is happy. You're no different. You can't be happy unless *all* of you is happy. When the different parts of you are pulling you in different directions, you have to feel miserable. Don't you see?"

I shrugged, showing my indifference, but he was not about to be put off. "You're in conflict right now and it feels rotten, doesn't it? A part of you is excited because something in this makes sense. But another part of you doesn't want to hear it, so you feel irritated and defensive. Call it whatever you want but you're not happy. Well, am I right?" he asked.

---

> **"Don't you see? You can't be happy unless *all* of you is happy. When the different parts of you are pulling you in different directions, you have to feel miserable."**

---

He was right. I knew he was right. I knew I should have been excited at the discovery, but I was feeling irritated and that took priority over any of his "revelations." I wanted to drop the whole thing. I felt as if on one level I was saying "yes, yes" and on another I just wanted him to go away. My professional training in psychology had taught me that conflict was at the seat of a great deal of unhappiness and that people would do a lot to avoid it. Still, I just didn't want to admit that he *might* be right.

Then the most astonishing thing happened. As I began to think about his idea—about his theory that parts of me were literally at war with each other—I became aware of something that had tortured me for years and that had kept me from truly enjoying the pride and joy of my weight loss.

---

**For the first time, I heard a voice inside my own head teasing me without mercy. I felt ugly and ashamed. I was being ridiculed and judged by people who were long gone and, until that very moment, I never knew it.**

---

For the first time, I heard a voice inside my own head teasing me mercilessly. "Pig, pig. Do a jig. Smelly, belly, big fat pig." I knew that I had been carrying around this taunt inside my own mind since I was a child. Of course I was unhappy. Though I had lost weight, and although to all the world I was slim, inside my head was living a six-year-old who was calling me names as so many other children had done. It was negating all the joy and pleasure that my new life had to offer.

My mind was telling me I "should" be happy and my body felt good, but my feelings were in desperate trouble. I felt ugly and ashamed. I was being ridiculed and judged by people who were long gone and, until that very moment, I never knew it.

Maybe Richard's "conflict" idea had something to it. I looked over the past week to see if there were instances when my mind or my body or my feelings were "in conflict" versus "in agreement" and if that made any difference in my happiness. I thought over each of the examples: I had been happy when I did a favor for an old friend for whom I had a great deal of affection. Well, that went along with the notion that when all parts of me were in agreement, I was happy. I remember that, at the time, I had wanted to help her out and that I had thought that it would be nice to do so. All of the parts of me, my mind, body, and feelings were in harmony, and I felt content.

I looked at another example: When I told my inconsiderate co-worker exactly what I thought, I felt good and, in fact, all of me was, once again, in agreement. My body was aching to let the feelings out, my feelings were overflowing, and my mind said that there would be no serious repercussions. The boss liked him less than I did and I knew I wouldn't get in trouble for speaking my mind. No conflict there. And, in fact, I had felt good. Hmmm. "This idea looks promising," I thought.

I decided to put Richard's conflict idea to the test. I looked for other examples, half-hoping to disprove his theory. When I received a good mark on a paper for school, my mind said that I had worked hard and I wanted the confirmation that I had done well. I worked hard; I deserved a good grade; I received a good grade. No conflict, no unhappiness.

When my good grade had failed to make me feel good, my mind had been saying that I had not worked hard enough on the paper and that I didn't deserve a good grade—although my feelings told me that I wanted to "get away with something." My feelings and my mind were in conflict and, in the end, the good grade didn't lead to good feelings. The essential parts of me were not in agreement; they were in conflict and, yes, I had been unhappy.

---

**A new feeling surged through me. For the first time in my life, I knew I was truly in control. I understood my feelings and, for once, things made sense. I knew what to do and how to do it.**

---

A new feeling surged through me. For the first time in my life, I knew I was truly in control. I understood my feelings and, for once, things made sense. I knew what to do and how to do it. If happiness was to be mine, I was going to have to work out the conflicts that existed between my mind, my body, and my feelings. Holding in my emotions, trying to avoid certain thoughts, ignoring my body's needs—none of these allowed me to be happy.

It seemed so obvious: In order to be happy, *all* the parts of me had to be in agreement. I could try to pretend that I wasn't angry, I could attempt to fake affection, I could persuade the outside world of many things—in other words, I could put on a great show, but in order to reach happiness inside myself, I could not lie to myself. I had done it for so long that a part of me wondered if I would even be able to tell the real from the fake. Somehow I trusted that I would. I was going to have to give up being the "good girl" and holding all of my real feelings inside. It was simple and it was clear, and, yet, I had been trying to avoid it for years.

Now began a task that would take several years of very hard work—to let go of the pain, fear, self-blame, and doubt that often caused my Circle of Success to break apart in conflict.

## Success Defined

---

**Success is knowing, without conflict, what you want—and then, getting it.**

---

I had always known that success meant different things to different people. Some people defined it as money, some as fame, some as love. Some had all of these and were still unhappy. Now I understood why. Success is knowing, without conflict, what you want—and then, getting it.

## The Facts and the Fury

*Rachael Continues:*

Five years had passed. Years marked by deep, honest, and difficult self-examination. Years of facing the unfinished anger left over from past relationships, of coming to grips with the many, many wrongs that had been done to me—the cruel words, the selfish betrayals, the subtle, and not-so-subtle, abuse.

The day was cold and crisp. Richard and I had just completed taping the "Sally Jessy Raphael Show." Each of us, in turn, had told our stories to the cameras and the audience: the years of shame, self-doubt, self-blame, abuse. We shared our before-and-after pictures, our pain, and our tears with a caring host and a wonderful audience. We spoke with pride and joy of our new lives and those of the carbohydrate addicts on our diet. We shared triumphant examples of living without weight concerns, hunger, or struggle. Who could ask for more?

Sally Jessy had embraced us, the producer loved us, the audience identified with us, and listeners wanting to know where to get *The Carbohydrate Addict's Diet* lit up the phone lines like a Christmas tree. We were sure to hit the *New York Times* best-seller list and hundreds of thousands of people would get the benefit of our experience. Certainly, we were a whopping success in every sense of the word!

Yet, even as the applause still rang in our ears, the looks that we exchanged with each other told us that something was "not quite right." Politely, we spent some time talking with the waiting fans and then headed for a nearby coffee shop.

I remember that, as we walked to a table, I couldn't contain myself. "Doesn't it bother you?" I demanded of Richard as we walked through the crowded restaurant. "They're missing it. All anybody talks about is weight loss, as if that's all there is. As if that's the end of it. It's as if, after you lose the weight, everything is supposed to be okay. You've lost the weight, now everything is great. But it's *not* great. It's just the beginning and nobody seems to want to know about all of the rest." We sat down.

I was nearly shouting and I knew it. The feelings of betrayal and the need to be understood were crushing my chest. Richard took my hand, ordered coffee so we wouldn't be thrown out of the restaurant, and squeezed my fingers reassuringly while he attended to the waitress.

I never gave him a chance to respond. "I mean it's not like my life didn't change. You know it did. But at the same time, it didn't. It was only the beginning. Some of the toughest fights were still to come. Why doesn't anybody want to know about those?"

Richard looked sad. "I know, but you have to understand how they're seeing it. When you look at a 165-pound weight loss like yours, that's all you focus on. I don't think they're to blame."

Richard hesitated and corrected himself before I had a chance to attack. "No, I take that back. I think it's much more than that. I think it's typical of the whole problem with society. When they see someone who's overweight, the only thing they see is the weight, and if someone loses it, all they see is the weight loss. That's the only thing they care about and, somewhere in between, the person inside gets lost in the shuffle. You're absolutely right. It's terrible. Only the weight matters to them. Whether they're talking then or now all they are looking at is the weight. It's as if all that you are is dependent on that one fact."

I swear, at that moment, no one could ever love anybody more than I loved him. He truly understood my feelings and put them in words that I will never forget. The coffee and my tears came at the same time. He asked for more napkins and poured some milk into my coffee.

---

**I put up with this for twenty-five years! Twenty-five years of believing that there was something really wrong with me. Twenty-five years of people telling me that I didn't want to lose weight "badly enough" or telling me that I was self-destructive or suicidal.**

---

I blew my nose and tried to stop crying, but as I took a cup of coffee, tears slid down my cheeks. "I put up with this for twenty-five years! Twenty-five years of believing that there was something really wrong with me. Twenty-five years of people telling me that I didn't want to lose weight 'badly enough' or telling me that I was self-destructive or suicidal. Suppose we had never discovered carbohydrate addiction? I'd still be somewhere all alone and blaming myself. And now, even though we understand what's causing the problem, even though we know how to correct it, half the time they still miss the point."

Richard's face looked tired and troubled, but he didn't try to get me to stop or deny what he knew was true. "Carrying the extra pounds are the least of it. It's the blame and the shame that other people put on you. The weight is nothing compared to how you know other people are judging you. You know, I used to want to live in Italy so that my weight wouldn't be a problem. They used to like heavy women there. But, apparently, they've changed their views and I wasn't really about to leave everything and everybody I knew so . . ."

My voice trailed off but I felt as if something in me had opened up. Finally, I was saying things that I had never allowed myself to admit to anyone. I took a breath and continued. "After I lost the weight, everyone—including me—expected me to be happy. All the blame and shame was supposed to vanish; all the self-righteous advice and wrongful accusations were supposed to be forgotten. Somehow, it was expected that I would be grateful and gracious and say, 'It's okay. I'm fine now. So what if everybody's advice was wrong all along. It's okay. So what if people made me feel like I was to blame for something that wasn't my fault. No problem. So what if I still carry the scars of self-doubt and self blame. I'll just take the years of suffering, denial, and abuse and be quiet about it. It's all right now so I won't mention it again. I'll be good and never speak of it again.'"

---

**After I lost the weight, everyone—including me— expected me to be happy. All the blame and shame was supposed to vanish; all the self- righteous advice and wrongful accusations were supposed to be forgotten.**

---

"Why don't they see, it simply doesn't work like that? A person doesn't just shrug their shoulders and walk off, happily ever after, off into the sunset." I stopped, looked up into Richard's caring face, reminded myself that he had gone through the same thing, softened my voice, and continued.

"We know what to do now, but it took both of us working together and years and years of hard work to free ourselves. And that was with both of us helping each other. Suppose you hadn't come along." My heart sank at the thought. "After all, look at some of the people in our groups. . . ."

Face after face came to mind, each with its own story, each with its own baggage. Once we had discovered and charted our own new territory, we were able to share it, in simple and easy terms, with others. Now, for several years, we had been working on a one-on-one level with our dieters at the Carbohydrate Addict's Center. We had been able to help them to cope with the remnants of the years of anguish and deprivation. We had helped them to find the freedom and happiness that comes from the mind, body, and feelings working in harmony. But as the demand for our help became greater, time became more and more of a problem.

We knew, then, that it was time to share with others the steps we had taken and the secrets we had uncovered (often by trial and error) that had led us to true feelings of success, to lives filled with joy, excitement, and, at the same time, peace of mind. From that moment this book was conceived, we wanted it to be the most loving, sensitive, and effective book that anyone had ever written. Our audience was (and is) very precious to us.

---

**Carbohydrate addicts live alone in a world that does not understand their addiction and which wrongly accuses, judges, and blames them.**

---

The emotional and psychological scars that carbohydrate addicts bear are equal-opportunity burdens; they span all weight levels, including those who had little or no weight to lose. The self-blame and self-doubt are shared by all ages and all backgrounds. Men and women alike have one common experience. If they are carbohydrate addicted, they have lived alone in a world that does not understand their addiction, and often they, too, have come to believe that they are to blame for their cravings and, in many cases, for their struggle with their weight.

The two of us finally realized that we had a common, physical addiction that bound us to other carbohydrate addicts. From that day, it became our shared mission to help relieve our fellow carbohydrate addicts of the blame that others had placed upon them so that we all might be free, together.

# CHAPTER 4

# Your Personal Circle of Success

Your Circle of Success is made up of three essential parts: your mind, body, and feelings. When the three parts of your Circle of Success are working together, they lead to success in terms of achievement, freedom, and happiness. When they are in conflict, you will experience loss of control, frustration, sadness, or hopelessness.

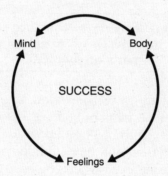

## The Essential Parts of Your Circle of Success

Your Circle of Success is made up of three basic parts: your mind, your body, and your feelings.

## The Crucial Connection

*No part of your Circle of Success stands alone.* Each part of your Circle of Success is strongly affected by the other parts. Taken together, they affect your ability to control your life and to get things done. Most important, they influence your feelings of freedom and happiness. When they are in harmony, you feel happy, you are able to act competently, and you feel confident. When they are in conflict, however, you feel torn apart, you no longer feel in control of your actions and life, and you may blame yourself.

Many of us know the old adage, "It's hard to be happy when your feet hurt." It's true. No matter how well things may be going, if you feel physically uncomfortable, you can't enjoy yourself. Even if something especially good happens to you and your mind is saying that you should be happy, if your body is in discomfort or pain, you simply don't *feel* happy. In a similar way, you may feel physically well, but if you are worried about something, you simply don't feel happy or free. Each part affects, and is affected by, the other two.

---

**Some people may try to convince you, often
for their own purposes, to ignore essential
parts of yourself.**

---

Some people may try to convince you, often for their own purposes, to ignore essential parts of yourself. "Don't worry!" they will tell you. "There's nothing to be upset about" or "Don't pay attention to it, it will go away." But your mind and body and feelings will not be silenced so easily, and even when you have done your best to ignore what they are trying to tell you, you will not rest easy until all parts of you are in harmony.

## Your Circle of Success in Harmony

For success and happiness, all three parts of the Circle must act together, pushing toward the center of the Circle. When they work together, they produce a greater push toward success than any one part could ever achieve alone. Like the instruments in a practiced orchestra producing a beautiful sound, the three parts of your Circle are in harmony when they are in agreement. You've experienced what harmony is like when you've seen a person or a team completely committed to a goal. Nothing, nobody, stands in their way. They don't feel conflict about what they want. They do not spend anguished moments first going in one direction, then another. They are not afraid of making a decision. They are not afraid of making a mistake. They are like pure energy and they are content in their work, no matter how demanding it may be.

---

**You may have experienced harmony yourself or you may have seen it in others. It is exciting, literally breathtaking. It is control at its best— without worry, fear, or doubt. It is true happiness.**

---

You may have experienced harmony yourself at certain times in your life. There may have been moments when you knew exactly what you wanted and found that your actions yielded the results you desired. It may have been a goal for yourself or for someone else. But, in any case, you knew the joy of being directed, unswerving, and content. Even if you have never seen nor experienced harmony of all parts of your Circle, chances are that you can almost imagine it, even as you read this paragraph. It is exciting, literally breathtaking. It is control at its best—without worry, fear, or doubt. It is true happiness . . . and that is what attaining your Circle of Success, and this book, are all about.

Here are all the parts of your Circle of Success working together, in harmony.

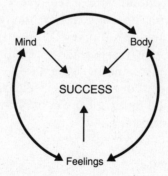

When all parts of your Circle are working together, in harmony, the absence of conflict allows you to experience a sense of purpose and, with it, the likelihood of success.

---

**The ability to know what you want, and to get what you want, may escape you right now, but once you learn how to reach your own harmony, it will help you to control your life and lead you to personal achievement, freedom, and happiness.**

---

The ability to know what you want, and to get what you want may escape you right now. You might not know how to capture that feeling of harmony at this moment, but we have found that bringing your Circle of Success into harmony is a skill that can be learned—easily and joyfully. Few of us come to it naturally, but once you learn how to reach your own harmony, it will help you to control your life and lead you to personal achievement, freedom, and happiness. We have done it. So have hundreds of thousands of others. So can you. Yes, you can.

## Your Circle of Success in Conflict

When any of the three parts of your Circle of Success are in conflict, you are pulled away from your center. You have experienced the result of conflict within your Circle every time you have seen your mind start to bring up a concern or worry and pull you away from a feeling of peace or happiness. You may have been feeling fine, doing the work that you wanted to get done, or relaxing and enjoying yourself. Along comes a thought or a comment from someone else, and suddenly, your mind and feelings are in conflict. You feel upset and you can't throw it off. Suddenly, in that moment, your peace and happiness are gone.

---

**Learning how harmony and conflict affect you
will help you to recapture your motivation,
freedom, and happiness. You will become less
vulnerable to your own negative thoughts as well
as to the opinions and criticisms of others.**

---

Learning about your own Circle of Success and how harmony and conflict affect you, will help you to recapture your motivation, freedom, and happiness, and make you less vulnerable to your own negative thoughts as well as to the opinions and criticisms of others.

Here are the three parts of your Circle of Success in conflict, pulling away from the center.

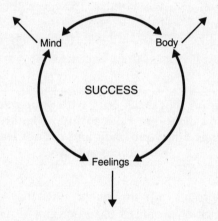

---

**As the parts of your Circle move away from the
center, you may feel confused, sad, anxious,
angry, frustrated, or irritable. You may find
that it is easy to lose your temper. Underneath,
you may feel hopeless.**

---

As the parts of your Circle move in opposite directions or away from the center, you will experience the thoughts and emotions associated with conflict. You may feel confused, sad, anxious, angry, frustrated, or irritable. When the parts are in conflict, you may find that it is easy to lose your temper. Underneath, you may feel hopeless. But the tears, fears, and outbursts are no more than the externalization of the conflict that you feel deep inside.

Each time one of the parts of your Circle pulls away from the center, it weakens the Circle; the greater the pull, the weaker the Circle. If the pull in the direction away from the center is strong enough, the Circle is broken and success, in terms of achievement, happiness, and freedom, cannot be achieved until, once again, all of the parts are in harmony.

Most programs that claim to aim at success at weight loss address only *one* of the three essential parts of your Circle. Some programs may focus on your mind. They provide you with "sensible" or "reasonable" steps to follow; they give you lists of food exchanges to trade, calories or portions to count or measure, cards to deal. They try to appeal to your sense of order and hope to sell you the illusion that their rules will give you control. However, their rules will only work in the short run because a program that deals only with your mind and gives you elaborate rules to follow ignores your feelings and your body and cannot, therefore, lead to permanent success.

---

**A program that deals only with your mind and gives you elaborate rules to follow ignores your feelings and your body and cannot lead to permanent success.**

---

Programs that focus only on your feelings may offer pep talks or inspirational stories or promises of future glory. They hope to sway you with emotion, knowing full well that any success you achieve will be temporary at best. Other programs, which concentrate only on the body (physical) component of your Circle of Success, may make up elaborate exercise regimens. They may issue "one-size-fits-all" recommendations related to exercise and try to keep you busy with so many minutes of physical activity or so many sit-ups. These programs fail to attend to your particular body's needs, to your metabolic level, and to your lifestyle. They do not address your feelings or your concerns. They do not take into account your preferences, lifestyle, and time demands.

In the end, no matter how disciplined you are and how hard you try, the chances are 49 to 1 that these programs will fail. And these very programs will blame you for their own failure. A few of the programs may combine two of the essential parts of the Circle, but they miss the essential combination of all three parts working together, and they are bound to fail in helping you to achieve an ongoing *successful* life. It is the interplay of your mind, body, *and* feelings, working together, that will bring about your success in terms of achievement, freedom, and happiness.

---

**Immediate or long-term failure is not the result of *your* lacking willpower, but is often the direct result of a program that does not give attention to all the parts that make up the very special person that we call *you*.**

---

Programs that do not address all three parts of your Circle of Success lead to conflict between the essential parts of your Circle. When they do not help you out of conflict, you are likely to feel anxious, frustrated, irritable, or sad. You may be very hard on yourself, or others. You may doubt your abilities, be fearful of making mistakes, or distrust yourself or friends. These are telltale signs that your Circle of Success is being broken by disharmony. But failure is not the result of *your* lacking willpower, but rather is the result of a program that does not give attention to all the parts that make up the very special person that we call *you*.

Carbohydrate addicts, in particular, are vulnerable to conflict because, whether or not they know it, carbohydrate addicts have a physical imbalance, *hyperinsulinemia*, which causes them to crave starches, snack foods, or sweets. Carbohydrate addicts' bodies are almost always in conflict with their thoughts and feelings. Because of their overabundance of insulin, they often feel compelling or recurring food cravings pushing them, against their desire, to eat. It is hard to be happy, or to keep up your motivation, or to stay in control, when your body is signaling you that you are hungry.

For the carbohydrate addict there is no peace. If we have just completed a meal, and for the moment we are not hungry, our minds tell us that we should *not* have eaten. We are worried about the consequences of our food splurge on our health or our weight.

We may be blaming ourselves for losing control. It's really hard to enjoy a sandwich when you think that you might be killing yourself.

For the carbohydrate addict, as for anyone, success, happiness, and freedom come when the Circle (and the harmony between the essential parts) remains unbroken, when they are all moving toward the center.

When all of the parts of your Circle are in agreement, you "naturally" feel good. One example of all the parts working in harmony might come when you are hungry and you know that it's okay to eat what you want and so you feel good about eating. Another example might be when you are not eating because you are not hungry and you feel good about that. In each case, your mind, your body, and your feelings are in harmony.

Success, in the form of peace or contentment, came, in the first example, with enjoying the food, and in the second example, with refraining from it. The definition of success changes depending on what all of the parts of you want. When the parts of your Circle are in conflict, so are you. When they are in harmony, so are you. Sounds simple but too good to be true? Well, it is simple and as so many have proven, and most assuredly, it's *not* too good to be true.

## Your Unique Circle of Success

In the Experiences that follow, you will learn a great deal about *your* own Circle of Success. Your feelings, your thoughts, the way your body reacts, are all essential elements in making *you* happy. What makes another person happy, what they define as success, is not yours. You are a unique individual. You are the sum total of a lifetime of experiences, joys, disappointments, attainments, achievements, and losses. You have a right to seek happiness and define success in your own terms.

---

**We are not concerned with what others think that you "should" do. This is your time. We are concerned with you being *you.* It is time to realize the happiness that is rightfully yours.**

---

We are not concerned with what others think that you "should" do. This is your time and we are interacting with you. Most of us tend to be "good" more often than not. We are concerned with you being *you*. Outside of doing anything that is illegal or will cause physical harm to another, we seek those actions that will bring you happiness.

Most of us put off seeking ourselves and our own happiness. We give to others in hopes that it will make us happy. Our lives slip away like sand through our fingers. We act as if we have all the time in the world. We don't. This is your moment. This is your life. You can make it what you want. Don't put it off one more day. Your life will slip away before you get a chance to live it. You have a right to be happy and now is the time. There will never be a time without worry or conflict or demands. Do it now. If not now, when?

Together, in the coming chapters, we will explore your unique Circle of Success and help you to realize the happiness that is rightfully yours.

# PART II

# Your Body: The Journey Within

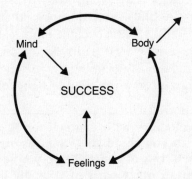

## A Guide to Your Journey

Have you ever had a "good breakfast" only to find that you were hungry before lunch? Do cravings or hunger pull you away from a diet that you really want to stay on? Do you find that when you eat a little bit of some foods you are unable to keep yourself from going back for more . . . and more?

In each of these instances, you have experienced your *body* pulling apart your Circle of Success. Your mind may have attempted to pull you toward success by reminding you how much you wanted to control yourself; your feelings may have tried to push you toward success by shaming or blaming you; or both might have been ominously silent, overpowered by your body's powerful need for satisfaction.

---

**We have long been taught to blame ourselves
whenever we lose control of our eating rather
than to look for a physical cause.**

---

When our body pulls us away from our Circle of Success, we wrongfully blame our mind or our feelings. We have long been taught by those around us to blame ourselves whenever we lose control of our eating, rather than to look for a physical cause. "She has no willpower." "He's killing himself, but what can you do?" "She just doesn't want to be thin badly enough." All of these reflect society's *incorrect* assumptions about what leads most people to fail at diets.

Science and medicine have long known that most overweight people have clear-cut physical differences that compel them to crave carbohydrates and to gain weight more easily than others. It would have been nice if science had won out long before this but, unfortunately, self-righteously blaming the victim has proved a great deal more satisfying and more profitable than rescuing the victim.

---

**Do you feel angry with yourself for "giving in"?
Do you wish you could stick to your diet but still
find yourself "out of control"? Do you see yourself
"in control" of other parts of your life but unable
to gain control of this one part of your life?**

---

If you have been blaming yourself for losing control of your eating and would like to see if you might have a physical problem that's influencing you, there's an easy way to tell the difference. Let's see if you have the following telltale signs: Do you feel angry with yourself for "giving in"? Do you wish you could stick to your diet but still find yourself "out of control"? Do you see yourself "in control" of other parts of your life but surprisingly unable to gain control of this one part of your life? If so, chances are you are experiencing the essential parts of your Circle of Success in conflict. Your body (and *not* your mind or your feelings) are pulling your Circle of Success apart and pushing success beyond your grasp.

Most of us are not used to paying attention to the messages that our bodies give. How many times have you put off going to the bathroom because you had something "more important" to do? Or been hot or cold but have not taken the time to attend to your needs until you felt physically ill or unable to work? The tendency to ignore our bodies' messages is especially strong when we are dieting. We have been told that we should use our minds and wills to overcome what our bodies want—not to satisfy them or, at best, to satisfy them only a little. This is the attitude of most weight-loss programs and it leads to their 98 percent failure rate. In contrast, we have found that it is only by listening to our bodies, by correcting the imbalances that lead to increasingly strong cravings, by normalizing our physical responses—that we have been able to succeed and, most important, maintain our success.

Learning about our bodies has brought us a great many surprises. It is humbling to learn that you have a physical addiction to carbohydrates. It is startling to learn that much of what we have long attributed to being "irritable" or "out of sorts" is, in fact, related to physical discomfort—discomfort that we may no longer pay attention to. It is enlightening to learn that often our bodies carry important messages that cannot, will not, be ignored, and that when we do ignore them, we suffer for it.

Your body is an essential part of your Circle of Success. Its needs must be attended to. If you try to ignore the messages your body gives you, eventually you are sure to fail. Mother Nature has the final word!!

---

**You may not be used to listening to your body.
You probably have simply demanded that it
perform for you, giving it little attention unless it
was so sick that it could not produce.**

---

You may not be used to listening to your body. You probably have simply demanded that it perform for you, giving it little attention unless it was so sick that it could not produce. The voice with which it may speak to you is probably soft and unsure. Like a child no one listens to, it has lost confidence and rarely speaks up unless it is desperate. Don't yell at yourself! Don't be impatient. Give yourself time to explore, learn, take chances, discover.

Most of us listen more to other people than to our own bodies. We don't take a nap unless we've "earned it" and we "have time." We eat the foods "most people eat." We feel guilty or secretive if we do what we want rather than what we think is expected of us. We become strangers to our own bodies or, at best, angry parents who put up with the demanding child we call our physical self. This leads us to unhappiness and failure.

Contrary to the pictures of the successful executive who is a workaholic, most truly successful people listen to what their bodies desire and indulge their physical needs. Success depends on taking the time you need to listen to yourself. Your body is a wonderful gift. It is your friend. Give it the respect and attention it deserves. It holds clues that will lead to your happiness and success. Don't bully or ignore it. Listen to what it is trying to tell you; if it is out of balance, correct the cause of the imbalance. Help your body to become normal—don't blame and punish it (and yourself).

# CHAPTER 5

# What Your Body Is *Really* Saying

Make a through study of the nature of the body which you would endeavor to heal.

—Hippocrates

## A Body Without a Wisdom of Its Own

*Richard:*

The signals that a carbohydrate addict's body is sending may be confusing. On the one hand it may say that you are full, even stuffed, after a large meal—and at the same time you still feel less than complete or satisfied. You may be aware that you have had "enough" to eat, but your body may be craving more.

---

**If I had listened to what my body was telling me, I would have heard demands for Oreos by the pound and ice cream by the gallon. *My body had no wisdom*. The more I gave it, the more it wanted.**

---

There are some diet "experts" who speak about the "wisdom of the body." "Just relax," they say. "Let your body speak to you. It will tell you what it needs." That never worked for me. If I had listened to what my body was telling me, I would have heard demands for Oreos by the pound and ice cream by the gallon. *My body had no*

**65**

*wisdom*. It was not "thirsting after calcium" or "potassium" or "fiber." It only knew the rule of insatiable demand. The more I gave it, the more it wanted.

My body wanted carbohydrates: bread, pasta, chocolate, cakes, cookies, potato chips. And it never seemed to get enough. I could eat until I felt I would burst. If, in its wisdom, my body wanted something, I would gladly have given it—but it wanted and wanted and wanted and was rarely, if ever, satisfied.

---

**I was hungry when I didn't eat
and miserable when I did.**

---

Almost all my life, I was hungry when I didn't eat and miserable when I did. One bite was too many and a thousand were not enough. I would eat until I fell asleep but, awake, I could find no peace.

Some bodies may provide their owners with some special kind of wisdom, but the carbohydrate addict's body is held captive by a physical addiction. When we say that you should listen to your body we mean that you should look for telltale signs of carbohydrate addiction and listen to your body's call for help. That does not mean that you should "give in" and indulge your every whim. Consider a situation in which you are caring for a young child who is tired and cranky. He demands one thing after another. You know he's exhausted but he won't lie down and go to sleep. You will quickly become frustrated if you listen to his demands. Instead, you step back and get some perspective on the situation. "He's exhausted," you tell yourself. "And he doesn't know enough to lie down and go to sleep." You probably put him down for a nap against all his protests; and, after some fussing, he's sleeping like an angel.

---

**The carbohydrate addict's body is like an
overtired child: there is no satisfying it. The more
you give in, the greater the demands.**

---

The carbohydrate addict's body is like an overtired child: there is no satisfying it. The more you give in, the greater the demands. If something is pleasing, it's temporary at best. For the carbohydrate addict, the power and drive to eat is, at times, literally overwhelming. At other times, it may be surprisingly manageable. Most diets will tell you to ignore strong impulses to eat . . . and eat . . . and eat. We say that these are important messages. They tell you that your body is not in balance and needs help. We are not recommending that you give in to those desires, but we think that the fact that you may have a physical problem that causes you to crave carbohydrates and to lose control must be addressed and made right. Then, and only then, will the cravings, hunger, self-blame, and weight problems become a thing of the past.

Together we will explore some of your past experiences with hunger and cravings and learn to recognize which are the result of your body's addiction to carbohydrates. Later in this book, we'll explore how your mind and your feelings influence your body's addictive response.*

## Your Body's Messages from the Past

### EXPERIENCE #1: SILENT SHOUTS, SOFTENED CRIES

Find a private, comfortable place and *sit* down and close your eyes. Do *not* lie flat.

Imagine yourself as an infant. You are alone in a crib in an empty room. You are hungry . . . and helpless. You start to cry. No one comes. You cry louder. Still, no one appears. The hunger intensifies. It hurts. You cry louder. Listen to your own screams. Let your thoughts come through. Listen to them.

What are you saying in your mind? _____

_____

_____

*Please note:* More details on reducing your hunger, cravings, and weight, together with a 17-item detailed test for carbohydrate addiction, appear in *The Carbohydrate Addict's Diet*.

Were you angry? Were you afraid? What were you feeling?

_____

_____

_____

_____

_____

Go back to your thoughts once again. Go back to you as the child alone, crying in the room. Let the intensity build once again. Now, complete your story in any way that you like.

What happened? Did someone come? Did they feed you?

_____

_____

_____

_____

_____

_____

How do you feel now? Are you relaxed or tense? Are you alert or groggy? Are you hungry?

_____

_____

_____

Now move to a flat, comfortable surface. Lie down.

If your story ended with your being lovingly fed, go back to that scene and bring yourself fully into it once again. Feel the warmth of the moment and, if you like, fall asleep to it.

If your story did not end in a nurturing way, go back and bring it to a nurturing, loving conclusion. Allow yourself to be fed, cuddled, and loved. Feel the warm milk nurture you and sustain you. Give yourself to the moment. Breathe deeply and let the feelings out.

Did you fall asleep? If so, write down any dreams you had or feelings that you had or that still linger. Take time to let the thoughts or feelings come through.

_____

_____

_____

_____

_____

What do you think these dreams or feelings may have been about?

_____

_____

_____

If you did not fall asleep, what thoughts crossed your mind?

_____

_____

_____

_____

Did you find it difficult to let go and be nurtured or did you openly welcome the food (or, perhaps, both)?

_____

_____

_____

_____

## Your Body's Messages Today

### EXPERIENCE #2: THE SIGNS OF CARBOHYDRATE ADDICTION

After nine years of experience we have learned to recognize the carbohydrate addict's repeated, predictable responses to food and hunger. Chances are, you're probably pretty sure that you are a carbohydrate addict, but let's observe your body's responses to food and hunger together and "scientifically" see how you rate as a carbohydrate addict.

GENERALIZED HUNGER
Generalized hunger is a strong urge for food of _any_ kind.
Generalized hunger occurs after you haven't eaten for a long period of time.
It passes in a little while, though it will reappear later.
"I'm _starving!_" best describes the experience of generalized hunger.
When you experience generalized hunger, you will probably eat just about anything that's put in front of you.
Close your eyes and try to remember what it has feels like to experience generalized hunger.

On a scale of 1–10, how hard is this hunger to control? _____

How often do you have this hunger? _____

Is your generalized hunger stronger at some times than at others?

_____

_____

_____

When you feel generalized hunger, what foods do you want to eat?

_____     _____

_____     _____

_____     _____

_____     _____

_____     _____

CRAVINGS (SPECIFIC HUNGER)

Cravings describe a strong desire to eat a *specific* food or kind of food.

Generally, cravings don't disappear completely; they may lessen for a short time (often if you are busy or distracted), but when they reappear they will probably be even more intense.

In the carbohydrate addict, cravings appear the more often you eat a particular food. Cravings are often easier to control when you've had none of the specific food you crave rather than when you've had "just a little."

"I could really go for _____ " best describes the experience of cravings.

When you experience cravings, you seek out that particular food or food group, although you may compromise and eat something else. If you compromise and eat a food that you don't particularly crave, you remain unsatisfied.

Close your eyes and try to remember what cravings feel like.

On a scale of 1–10, how hard are cravings to control? _____

How often do you experience cravings? _____

Are your cravings stronger at some times than at others? _____

_____

_____

When you experience cravings, what foods do you want to eat?

Now, complete Experience #3 and see what your answers from both experiences indicate in the scoring section that follows.

## EXPERIENCE #3: ARE YOU A CARBOHYDRATE ADDICT?

Check off "Yes" or "No" to each of the following questions:

1. Do you experience cravings more often than you experience generalized hunger?                    YES \_\_\_ NO \_\_\_

2. Is it easier for you to control your generalized hunger than cravings?                    YES \_\_\_ NO \_\_\_

3. When you experience cravings, is it likely to be for some of the following foods: starches (like bread or pasta or rice), snack foods, and/or sweets?                    YES \_\_\_ NO \_\_\_

4. Do you find that your cravings increase when you have had some of the following: starches (like bread or pasta or rice), snack foods, and/or sweets? YES ___ NO ___

**SCORING YOUR RESPONSES:**

1. Generalized hunger is normal, and although cravings can be normal as well, when you experience cravings two to three times more often than generalized hunger, carbohydrate addiction is usually the cause. So look at your numbers and see if your cravings estimate is two to three times greater than your hunger estimate. If so, count this as a "yes" answer.

2. Carbohydrate addicts have a physically based hormonal imbalance (although they may not be aware of it) and, because of the imbalance, carbohydrate addicts often have a very hard time controlling their cravings. Most carbohydrate addicts tell us that they find generalized hunger much easier to control than cravings. The nonaddict finds that cravings are easier to control than generalized hunger. If you have a harder time controlling your cravings than your generalized hunger, count this as a "yes" answer.

3. The more often carbohydrate addicts have carbos the more they crave them. "I'm okay if I don't have any, but once I start, I can't stop" is a typical carbohydrate addict statement. If this describes you, count it as a "yes" answer.

4. Look at the foods that you have listed in the *craving* section of Experience #2. Have you listed a greater number of carbohydrate-rich foods (like breads, pasta and other starches, snack foods, fruit, and/or sweets) than all other foods put together? If so, count this as a "yes" answer.

5. Look at the foods that you have listed in the *hunger* section of Experience #2. Have you listed a greater number of carbohydrate-rich foods (like breads, pasta and other starches, snack foods, fruit and/or sweets) than all other foods put together? If so, count this as *two* "yes" answers.

**YOUR SCORE:**

A score of 2 or more "yes" answers to the preceding questions may indicate carbohydrate addiction. The greater the number of "yes" answers, the greater the chances that you are a carbohydrate addict, and most likely your body has been telling you so!

## Your Body's Messages in the Future

### EXPERIENCE #4: AN END TO DEPRIVATION

Your hunger, your cravings are real. They come from a physical part of you that lies at the very base of life itself. Most of us have come to associate our cravings and hungers with shame, blame, anger, and fear. Your hunger and desires are your life force, demanding sustenance and nourishment. It is life itself. It is you.

You have completed the first three Experiences in this chapter. Now it is time to let go of the hungry part of you that you have battled with in the past.

Tear the first three Experiences out of the book and destroy them. That's right, destroy them.

You may want to tear the Experiences into little pieces or burn them. Do not hesitate. It is part of your breaking free; it is an essential part of your healing. You don't need to remember your responses. You need to let them go. As we continue, chapter by chapter, we will replace this book with a Success folder—one that will guide you and help you in the future. It is time to leave behind the painful experiences of the past.

As you destroy each of the first three Experiences from your past and present, visualize your Circle of Success encircling you, feel the circle around you grow strong in harmony and say *out loud:*

"*I* will feed me. *I* will take care of me."

"My hungers are cries of life and I will honor them."

"I will give myself the things that I need so that I may be healthy and strong."

"If my body does not know what it needs, I will guide it."

"I will learn to recognize the difference between real hunger and addictive cravings."

"I will feed myself when I am hungry and lovingly guide myself to a life free of addiction."

"Deprivation is not my lot in life."

"I have a right to fulfillment and nourishment given with love and with tenderness."

"My body has been given to me in trust and I will care for it with love, with compassion, and with understanding."

Now take this page and put it in a new folder or envelope—this will become your Success folder. Other pages from other chapters will be added to it later.

Look at this sheet regularly and read it, saying out loud the words you need to hear to heal your body of the negative experiences of the past.

It is time to walk tall and proud into the future. Let the words on this page guide you.

# CHAPTER 6

# S.A.L.T.: Stressed? Angry?
# Lonely? Tired?

*Stress:* The capacity of a man is revealed only under stress and he may then be a splendid surprise to himself.
                      —*Consecratio medici*

*Anger:* To be angry with the right person and to the right extent and at the right time and in the right way—that is most difficult.           —*Nicomachean Ethics*

*Loneliness:* To feel alone when you are alone, that is one thing; to feel alone when you are not alone, that is another.
                      —Japanese proverb

*Tiredness:* Life is one long process of getting tired.
                      —Samuel Butler

## A Sexy but Incorrect Assumption

*Rachael:*

It amazes me that so many self-proclaimed diet experts assume that hunger is psychological, mental, or emotional in origin. "It's all in your head," they will tell you. "You eat because you are trying to fill other needs," they pronounce self-righteously. "You eat when you want love," says one. "You eat when you are upset," says another. "No, no. You eat when you are angry," proclaims a third. Another adds that "You eat when you are sublimating unacceptable desires or wishes."

It doesn't seem to matter to either news anchorpersons or to au-

77

thors or to some doctors or dietitians that science has long known that many of the people who have strong cravings simply have too much insulin. The news media find that it is far "sexier" simply to ignore the findings of decades of scientific work and go on assuming that anyone who has a weight problem should be blamed for their "lack of willpower." To make matters worse, many health professionals are influenced by the powerful but unknowing reports of the press.

Both Richard and I have lived with these assumptions, or more accurately, these accusations, all of our lives. Our research and our work, our success with hundreds of thousands of other carbohydrate addicts, is testimony to the fact that the claims and blames of "experts" are simply untrue.

Our personal lives, as well, contradicted the long-held assumptions that eating was psychological. Sure, both Richard and I eat when we're angry—and when we're sad—and when we have felt unloved—just as conventional wisdom says. But we have gone to the bathroom at these times as well. Does that mean that going to the bathroom is psychological, too?

---

**Some people may get hungry when they're emotionally upset, but they probably also get hungry when they're bored or when they don't want to tackle that pile of work.**

---

Some people may get hungry when they're emotionally upset, but if they take time to think about it, they will likely find that they probably also get hungry when they're bored or when they simply want to avoid a pile of work that's waiting to be done. We eat to reward ourselves, to fulfill ourselves, to relax, to celebrate, to put off other things, and, sometimes, for absolutely no reason whatsoever. Eating is not "all psychological," no matter what some people want to believe. There are nervous people who are thin and nervous people who are fat. There are carbohydrate addicts with lives full of stress and stressed nonaddicted people as well.

Study after study has failed to find a single "psychological" problem or "motivational" or "behavioral" profile that exists in those of us who battle weight and eating, but does not exist in the person who is naturally slim. Even the American Psychiatric Association no longer lists simple "obesity" as either a psychological or a behavioral problem. What's left? Biological—and many of us who have struggled with our weight knew it all along. For many people, the newspaper and magazine articles that hail the weight-gaining effects of anger and stress are a thinly veiled type of name-calling.

In our preliminary work at Mt. Sinai School of Medicine we have offered neither psychological nor motivational counseling to our carbohydrate addicts. Instead, we concentrated on changing the body's response to food, and we found unprecedented success by treating only "the physical" part of the problem. This confirmed that a biological problem lay at the base of most of the eating and weight difficulties of our dieters.

## The Stress Connection

In the first years of our research, one point still remained a mystery to us. We found that although many people reported that they felt hungrier when they found themselves "under pressure" or "stress" or when they "got depressed," others did not. Some said that these experiences were almost sure to bring about hunger or cravings, whereas others said that stress clearly did not affect their cravings. We were at a loss to explain the differences.

In order to try to understand what actually happened to our carbohydrate addicts under stress, we closely monitored each person's day-to-day experience of hunger and we came up with some startling results. Just as they reported, some of the people we studied were no more likely to crave carbohydrates when they were angry or stressed than they did at any other time. But for others, the difference in their cravings was astounding. For these carbohydrate addicts, stress, anger, tiredness, and loneliness set off incredibly strong desires for carbohydrate-rich foods.

---

**For some carbohydrate addicts, stress, anger, tiredness, and loneliness set off incredibly strong desires for carbohydrate-rich foods.**

---

Years of investigation have led us to understand that the hunger that some of our carbohydrate addicts experience under these conditions is the result of a *biological* connection between these "stressors" and a too great release of insulin. For these dieters, what used to be referred to as "psychological" is, in reality, the result of an error in their hormonal regulatory system. In other words, for some people, stress, anger, loneliness, and/or tiredness may start out as psychological but very quickly become physical.

---

**The impact of stress, anger, loneliness, and tiredness on a person's hunger and cravings is experienced differently by different people.**

---

Our professional work, and our personal lives as well, have repeatedly shown us that health professionals must learn to respect individual differences. The impact of stress, anger, loneliness, and tiredness on a person's hunger and cravings is experienced differently by different people. Some people under stress may barely notice any difference in their hunger or cravings, whereas others may be strongly affected.

For most of our *severe* carbohydrate addicts, stress, anger, loneliness, and tiredness—what we call *S.A.L.T.*—has no impact. The bodies of these carbohydrate addicts are so strongly pulled to carbohydrates already that increases in hunger or cravings by the four stressors literally go unnoticed. Adding stress to their bodies is somewhat like pouring a quart of water into the ocean; there is so much water there already that adding more makes little difference.

In contrast, for the moderate or the mild carbohydrate addict, the impact of stress, anger, loneliness, or tiredness (*S.A.L.T.*) can be quite devastating:

---

**Lisa gave her all and it took its toll.**

---

### Lisa's Story:

Lisa J. was in a high-pressure job. She worked on the floor of the New York Stock Exchange. She was relatively new to the business, but in her six months there, it had become clear to everyone that she was going to go far. She fought hard for her clients. She gave her all and it took its toll. In six months Lisa had gained more than 25 pounds. "I don't understand it," she told us. "Sure, I watched my weight before I came here, but it was nothing like this. I'm totally out of control. I used to tease my sister for not being able to control her eating. Now I stuff M&M's in my pockets so I have something to tide me over till lunch. I feel like I just can't get enough to eat. I'm always hungry."

Lisa's problem was getting worse, not better. "In the beginning, I knew it was stress. I knew the job was making me crazy and hungry at the same time. But it was okay—sort of. I would eat all week, sometimes uncontrollably (you should have seen me at night when I got home), but I would be very strict during the weekend and could usually take off some of the weight that I had put on all week. Now, I've totally lost control. Weekend, weekday, it doesn't matter. I'm always hungry and I can't get it under control. I don't want to give up my job, but I'm afraid that I'm just going to keep gaining weight. It doesn't feel like it's ever going to stop."

Within a matter of days we were able to help Lisa handle the stresses of her job without "going crazy over food." We put her on the Carbohydrate Addict's Diet, and helped her through the Experiences that follow. She found that she did not have to choose between controlling her eating and weight and her new career.

Today, four years later, she is a sleek, happy, and successful Wall Street broker.

## The Stress That Comes from Your Past

### EXPERIENCE #5: A FORCE TO BE RECKONED WITH

Read the following lines one by one. At the end of the paragraph, close your eyes and allow yourself to experience the feeling or remember the situation.

Think over the recent past. Try to remember a single incident when someone was demanding or expecting something from you. Maybe it was a time when you found yourself responsible for something or when you were trying hard to do something well or within a time limit. Or perhaps it was a moment when you were pressuring yourself. Close your eyes and remember where you were and what was happening.

What were others saying? What were you thinking? What were the demands on you? Try to hear the actual words.

_____

_____

_____

_____

_____

_____

_____

Now, close your eyes again and let yourself reexperience what you were feeling when you were under that stress. Let the experience come through. Don't hold your feelings back.

When we are under stress, different parts of our body may respond to the stress in different ways and to different degrees.

Some examples:

Your legs might feel "tight," "crampy," or even "relaxed."

You might have "pain" or a "sinking feeling" in your stomach.

You might have felt "weak," "warm," "cold," or any combination of these feelings, or others.

What were you feeling:

in your head? _____

in your neck? _____

in your shoulders? _____

in your chest? _____

in your back? _____

in your stomach? _____

in your arms or legs? _____

What would you have liked to say to others or, perhaps, to yourself?
Say it now. Out loud. Really let it out, then write it down here.

_____

_____

_____

_____

   Now, repeat what you would have liked to say but, this time, say
it over and over again until you feel the tension leave your body. Do
it until the stress is completely gone. It's vitally important to let go
of the demands of others (as well as the voices inside your head).
*Take the time to do this part of the Experience* even if it feels odd.
You may not be used to letting out the stresses you hold inside unless it bursts out in a rage, but you have the right to free yourself of
the stresses and demands that you, yourself, and others place upon
you in a controlled, deliberate way.

   Take a moment now to continue to repeat what you would have
liked to say. Write it or say it over and over, no matter how many
times it takes, until you feel no more emotion connected with it—no
more tension, no more pressure.

I would have liked to say _____

_____

_____

I would have liked to say _____

_____

_____

I would have liked to say _____

_____

_____

I would have liked to say _____

_____

_____

I would have liked to say _____

_____

_____

Hold onto these thoughts for now. We will use them at the end of the next Experience.

## The Anger That Comes from Your Past

### EXPERIENCE #6: THE FIRE THAT BURNS

Read the following lines one by one. At the end of the paragraph, close your eyes and allow yourself to experience the feeling or remember the situation.

Think over the past. Try to remember a single incident when someone or something made you furious. You may not have exploded at the moment, or you might not have even shown your anger, but you felt it just the same.

If it's hard to remember any situation that made you angry, you might find that you are hiding some of these feelings from yourself. If you are "one of those people who simply don't get angry," remember, instead, an incident that would have made anyone else furious.

In either case, close your eyes and remember where you were and what was happening.

What caused the anger? What were others saying? What were you thinking and saying?

_____

_____

_____

_____

_____

_____

_____

Now, close your eyes again and let yourself reexperience what you felt when you were in the anger-making situation. Let the feelings come through. Don't hold them back.

When we feel angry, different parts of our body may respond to the feelings in different ways and to different degrees.

Some examples:

Your legs might feel "tight," "crampy," or even "relaxed."

You might feel like kicking or running.

You might feel a lump in your throat.

You might have "pain" or a "sinking feeling" in your stomach.

You might have felt "weak," "hot," "cold," or any combination of these feelings, or others.

What were you feeling:

in your head? _____

in your neck? _____

in your shoulders? _____

in your chest? _____

in your back? _____

in your stomach? _____

in your arms or legs? _____

What would you have liked to say to others or to yourself? Say it now. Really let it out. Say it out loud, then write it down here.

_____

_____

_____

_____

Now, repeat what you would have liked to say but, this time, say it over and over again until you feel your body relax. Do this until the anger is completely gone. It's vitally important to let go of the anger that remains inside. Take the time to do this part of the Experience, even if it feels new.

We are not used to letting out the anger that we hold inside, but you have the right to be free of the anger that you have felt for so long. There are many things we would have liked to say or do.

I would have liked to: _____

_____

_____

I would have liked to: _____

_____

_____


I would have liked to: _____

_____

_____


I would have liked to: _____

_____

_____


I would have liked to: _____

_____

_____


Imagine, in detail, the action you would have liked to have taken or, aloud, say what you would have liked to say. Take the time to imagine the action or say the words until the feelings leave your body. How do you feel now:

     in your head? _____

     in your neck? _____

     in your shoulders? _____

     in your chest? _____

in your back? _____

in your stomach? _____

in your arms or legs? _____

Now let's compare the two Experiences. Think over the feelings of stress and the feelings of anger that you explored in the past two Experiences.

Stress and anger are different, but they can sometimes feel almost the same inside. Stress is a demand on us, from ourselves or others, to change; to do something more quickly or without error or both; to take on impossible tasks and to do them perfectly; or to do more of them than we are able. Stress points inward. Anger, on the other hand, points outward. Behind anger is your strong demand that a person or situation be different or change.

Yet, for many of us, stress and anger can feel pretty much the same. We can confuse them in the moment. Our bodies tighten, we want to strike out or yell but, more often than not, we hold it in. Or at least we think we hold it in. As most of us know, "it's not what you're eating; it's what is eating you" that can be a problem.

The anger or stress that resides within us can literally change the way our bodies respond. When we are feeling angry we may be much more prone to interpret mild requests as stressful, and when we are feeling stressed we are far more likely to respond with anger. It is important to separate your feelings of stress and anger so that one does not build on the other, for they can make us sick in more ways than one. They literally unbalance us and cause us "dis-ease."

One result of an imbalance can be an endocrine system that is no longer able to regulate food intake wisely. It is no wonder that we feel hungry and unsatisfied and that we seek something to right that imbalance.

Carbohydrates cause the body to produce the brain chemicals that soothe and relax us but, for the carbohydrate addict, this balance is temporary at best. Within a short time, the imbalance returns and the addictive cycle repeats . . . and repeats and repeats. The goal of this book, and our lives, is to take the feelings and thoughts that cause our bodies to crave carbohydrates and let them in, let them out, and let them go, and with the letting go, move on with our less-addicted lives.

Sometimes letting go of stress and anger can be relatively easy, and at other times it can be more difficult than you ever imagined. Stress tends to be a temporary experience, and a good night's sleep or some time and distance may help you to gain perspective. After you have had some rest, you might choose to calmly remove yourself from the situation that's causing you the stress or simply learn not to take the demands of others quite so seriously. But there are times when you may find yourself stuck in a situation and, try as you will, unable to disregard the demands being placed on you.

Getting rid of anger is especially hard, especially when you feel that you have been treated poorly, or worse, unfairly. You may say to yourself, "I'm not going to let him get away with that" or "Why should I put up with that?" and try to get the person to act in ways that are more appropriate. Certainly, whenever it is possible, change what you can, but changing some people, as you know, is simply impossible.

If you have tried to right a wrong and you find that you cannot, or if you know that to do so would not be a good choice, let go. Let go of trying to "make it right" and, most of all, let go of the feelings of being wronged or being misunderstood. Let in the awareness that this is simply something that you cannot change. The world is not always fair, and hard as it may be, we all must learn to live with it. It is a very, very difficult reality to accept. You want to make it right, but sometimes, no matter how hard you try, you just can't. That's when it's time to let go and move on with your life rather than wasting any more time or energy (conscious or unconscious) on it. In the pages that follow we will give you guidance and help in letting go of the stress and anger that can impact on your life and your weight.

Remember: Although you can't change what was, you can still move ahead and change what *will* be. That's where the real power to make things fair resides.

# The Loneliness That Comes from Your Past

EXPERIENCE #7: THE DEEPEST ACHE OF ALL

*Rachael:*

Loneliness has been a particularly strong feeling for me and has a great deal of meaning. When I look back at it now, it seems that, until I met Richard, I spent most of my lifetime alone. Even when I was with people, I still felt as if I was spending most of my time trying to please them or to understand them. I can count on my fingers the moments that I felt that a special someone really cared about me.

My loneliness was more than just a need for the company of others (though it was often that as well), but also the need to be cared for and . . . valued. I longed to be with someone who understood me and heard what I thought and felt. I ached to share my ideas, my insights, my hopes, my pain—all with someone who cared.

We live in a time when society says that it's okay to feel tired or sick or "out of sorts," but when it comes to loneliness, well, no one really talks about it. That means that when you are lonely, you probably don't talk about it much and, of course, that makes you feel more isolated and lonely.

Loneliness makes us human and compassionate. These tender feelings are important. They complement the stronger feelings that might otherwise make us a bit arrogant and demanding.

Now, it's time to bring them out. Think of a time when you felt truly alone, when you found yourself frightened or sad or longing for a particular person or just desired some company, in general. It might have been a special event that you would have liked to share with someone else, or it might have just been a time when you really needed someone to care. Close your eyes and remember where you were, what was happening, and what you were feeling and thinking.

_____

_____

_____

_____

_____

_____

When we are under lonely, different parts of our body may respond to those feelings in different ways.

Some examples:

> Your legs might feel "relaxed" or even "dead."

> You might feel "weepy" or have an "empty feeling" in your stomach.

> You might have felt "weak," "warm," "cold," or "disconnected" or numb or any combination of these feelings, or others.

What were you feeling:

in your head? _____

in your neck? _____

in your shoulders? _____

in your chest? _____

in your back? _____

in your stomach? _____

in your arms or legs? _____

What would you have liked to do or to say to others or, perhaps, to yourself? Say it now. Gently let it out. Say it first, then write it down here.

_____

_____

_____

_____

Now, repeat, in writing or by saying it, what you would have liked to say, but this time, repeat it over and over again until you feel the tension leave your body. Do it until the pain that remained is completely gone. Take the time to do this part of the Experience even if it feels unusual. We are not used to releasing the feelings we hold inside, but it's hard to trust others and yourself when those feelings remain.

I would have liked to say _____

_____

_____

I would have liked to say _____

_____

_____

I would have liked to say _____

_____

_____

I would have liked to say _____

_____

_____

I would have liked to say _____

_____

_____

Take a moment now to recall a time when you had a good friend, someone you were dating, or somebody in your family that you could trust, someone who understood and cared about you, someone with whom you could share your thoughts and feelings. Don't think about what has come and gone since that time, just remember them as they were back then.

Remember what it felt like to be you then—the freedom of being liked for who you were and cared for and valued.

Now let these feelings spread throughout your body and fill you.

## The Tiredness That Comes from Your Past

EXPERIENCE #8: A HUNGER FOR REST

*Richard:*

When I get tired, all of the negative thoughts and feelings I might be holding inside intensify. I feel irritable. Nothing seems right. Usually, I don't have the good sense to lie down. I push myself to keep going and, almost without fail, I get hungry.

Sometimes I feel like eating in order to reward myself for continuing to keep going in the face of exhaustion, but usually it is a simple matter of biology. My body literally hungers for sleep, but I keep pushing that hunger away. My blood sugar level dips and my body longs for bread or muffins, for a good bagel or a sandwich. I can barely think clearly; still I keep going. It is no surprise that, sooner or later if I don't get rest, I "give in" and eat.

Sometimes there are real reasons that I can't rest; I'm scheduled to teach a class at the medical school or my manuscript is due tomorrow. But sometimes I just don't value myself enough to take the time to give me what I need. It is easier and quicker to put some food in my mouth than to lie down for an hour.

Resting your body is important. You are not a machine used just to produce what is needed (and even a machine needs rest and maintenance). When you are tired you need to be able to recognize it and attend to it. The eating plan in *The Carbohydrate Addict's Diet* will help eliminate a great deal of your tiredness that may be due to what we call "carbohydrate fatigue." Other tiredness may be due to emotional strain or physical exhaustion. Even when you think that you "shouldn't" be tired, you may really need a rest. First, you must learn to pay attention to your tiredness; then, you must attend to it. Often, it will not really go away but will be converted into hunger or cravings. It's time to stop depriving your body of what it truly craves. When it's tired, let's give it rest.

Close your eyes and focus on what you are feeling.

Right now, are you feeling tired:

in your head? _____

in your neck? _____

in your shoulders? _____

in your chest? _____

in your back? _____

in your stomach? _____

in your arms or legs? _____

If you find that you are tired and you can take a nap or lie down and relax, *do it now.* If you can't lie down, close your eyes and relax in the most comfortable place you can find. If you are at work, close a door if possible. If there is no comfortable chair, lie down on the floor. If there is no private space, go to the bathroom. In any case, give yourself a few moments of rest. Eleanor Roosevelt used to swear that ten-minute naps were her key to survival. Even if you don't sleep, give yourself a well-deserved and long-awaited break.

During the next week, take time to schedule in rest times and extra sleep for yourself. Try it for one week and see how much better you feel. Make it a priority in your life. Just for one week! Once you experience how good it feels, give yourself the right to keep it as a personal priority.

## The Stress, Anger, Loneliness, and Tiredness That Influence Your Present

EXPERIENCE #9: WHAT'S YOUR S.A.L.T. LEVEL—ARE YOU STRESSED? ANGRY? LONELY? TIRED?

Now let's look at *you* and the way that your particular body responds to stress, to anger, to loneliness, and to tiredness. The chart which follows will help you to determine your particular S.A.L.T. level.

For two full days, fill in the appropriate lines on the chart that follows. Pick days that are different "kinds" of days for you—one that is busy (full of tasks) and one that is more leisurely (or as close to leisurely as you get). Perhaps a weekday and a Sunday if that's appropriate for you. They don't have to be two days in a row.

For each of these two days, pay careful attention to your urge to eat. Notice when you have either hunger or cravings. Anytime that you experience either hunger or cravings, stop what you are doing and fill in all the items on one line in the chart that follows. As long as you experience hunger or cravings, fill in the items on the chart, even if you don't actually eat anything. If the cravings or hunger remain for a half an hour, note the experience as an additional entry on the chart. Repeat the entry for each additional half hour it remains. Do not blame yourself for your hunger or cravings. Just note them on the chart. No one is judging you. This is simply a way to gather more information about your particular body and the way it responds, so that we can better help you.

Try to avoid telling yourself that you'll fill in your chart later. When you put off filling in your chart it is easy to forget the way you felt or what you were thinking. Take out your chart and fill in the columns as soon as you feel the urge to eat. This chart is an important map that will help guide us in charting your new life and success.

## S.A.L.T. DIARY

| Date | Time | Feeling Hunger or Cravings? | Food Desired (Most Desired First) |
|------|------|------------------------------|-------------------------------------|
|      |      |                              |                                     |
|      |      |                              |                                     |
|      |      |                              |                                     |
|      |      |                              |                                     |
|      |      |                              |                                     |
|      |      |                              |                                     |
|      |      |                              |                                     |
|      |      |                              |                                     |
|      |      |                              |                                     |
|      |      |                              |                                     |
|      |      |                              |                                     |
|      |      |                              |                                     |
|      |      |                              |                                     |
|      |      |                              |                                     |
|      |      |                              |                                     |
|      |      |                              |                                     |
|      |      |                              |                                     |
|      |      |                              |                                     |

| Feeling Stressed? | Feeling Angry? | Feeling Lonely? | Feeling Tired? |
|---|---|---|---|
|  |  |  |  |
|  |  |  |  |
|  |  |  |  |
|  |  |  |  |
|  |  |  |  |
|  |  |  |  |
|  |  |  |  |
|  |  |  |  |
|  |  |  |  |
|  |  |  |  |
|  |  |  |  |
|  |  |  |  |
|  |  |  |  |
|  |  |  |  |
|  |  |  |  |
|  |  |  |  |
|  |  |  |  |

Use the chart you filled out for two days and count up your
*S.A.L.T.* score. Count up only those entries for hunger or tiredness
that also had a check for either stress or loneliness or anger or tiredness.

DAY #1 (Work or task-filled day)
  Number of times you were:
  Hungry _____          Craving _____
  Number of times you were:
  Stressed: _____    Angry: _____
  Lonely: _____    Tired: _____
DAY #2 (Nonwork or more leisurely day)
  Number of times you were:
  Hungry _____          Craving _____
  Number of times you were:
  Stressed: _____    Angry: _____
  Lonely: _____    Tired: _____

Now, let's see what your answers tell us about you and your *S.A.L.T.*
responses:

DAY #1 (Work or task-filled day):
  Which did you experience more often: hunger or crav-
  ings? _____
  Did you find that you were more often stressed or an-
  gry or lonely or tired? _____
DAY #2: (Nonwork or more leisurely day)
  Which did you experience more often: hunger or crav-
  ings? _____
  Did you find that you were more often stressed or an-
  gry or lonely or tired? _____
What does your S.A.L.T. score tell you about yourself? (More
than one may apply.)

If you had a greater number of stress, anger, loneliness, or tiredness entries connected to cravings rather than to hunger:

You are showing a carbohydrate-addicted response to stress,
anger, loneliness, or tiredness.

If you had far more S.A.L.T.–related cravings on one day than on the other:

> Something in that day's particular environment appears to be stimulating an addictive response in you. You may already have a pretty good idea as to what it is, but if you aren't sure, repeat the exercise for two days under different conditions. For example, when your boss is in the office and again when he/she is on vacation, or when you and your children are getting along versus when you are not. If you see a consistent pattern of cravings during one condition and far fewer cravings during another, you may have uncovered an important trigger to your carbohydrate addiction.

If your number of S.A.L.T.–related cravings on both days were pretty much the same:

> You may be experiencing stress or tiredness or anger or a feeling of being separate and alone in *both* environments or you may be carrying the responses of one day into the other so that a boss that drives you crazy may trigger your short-tempered response to a spouse at home (or vice versa).
>
> If you can identify the specific trigger, try to eliminate it by removing it from your life or by changing your response to it. (We will offer lots of suggestions in the pages to come.) If you cannot identify the trigger or if it remains a problem, professional assistance may be necessary. Remember that in understanding that your emotions can trigger cravings, you are already far ahead of the game. Now you might need a little help in permanently removing that connection from your life.

If any one of the S.A.L.T. responses—stress, anger, loneliness, or tiredness—far outnumbers the others and is connected to cravings:

> Your body is demanding attention. Clearly you need take care of the problem, and yourself. The problem will not go away, and no matter what you tell yourself, it is taking its toll on your health or your happiness. Do not fool yourself into

thinking that you can ignore it. Look over the restoration recommendations in the last Experience in this book. Take the
actions you need to change your life. Addiction triggers can
be your body's cry for help.

If your cravings are connected to two of the S.A.L.T. responses
(for example, tiredness at work and anger at home):

Both triggers may reflect the same problem. Look for a common source that may be causing a ping-pong effect. Anger at
work, for instance, may simply be a reflection that you are
pushing yourself until you are exhausted. In that case, give
yourself the rest that you so badly need.

---

**Just as you might close your eyes to bright light,
you may react to stress (or anger or loneliness or
tiredness) by feeling the urge to eat.**

---

Your *S.A.L.T.* score details an important connection for you and
you alone; that is, your link between food and feeling. We are *not*
saying that your desire for food is "psychological," but rather that
your body is very complex and that it responds to what you feel and
think as well as to what is said and done to you. When you have intense feelings, there are chemical changes that occur in your body
and these, in turn, may influence your desire for food.

In some people, when thoughts or feelings get too intense, the
body responds by wanting food almost as if it were responding to
a reflex. Just as you might close your eyes to bright light, you may
find that you react to stress (or anger or loneliness or tiredness) by
feeling the urge to eat. This reaction is *not* a reflection of your willpower or your psychological health or how strong a person you are.
Your urge to eat or the cravings that you feel are simply the ways
that your particular body responds to those particular feelings.

It has long been assumed that whether or not you "give in" to
these feelings to eat reflects your commitment to your diet or your
drive to be successful, and that whether or not you can "control"
yourself shows how motivated you are. *We strongly disagree.* We
have found that whether or not you "give in" and eat is, in very

great part, determined by how strong your hunger or cravings are as compared with others.

Richard and I are the same people we were 200 pounds ago. We have the same willpower and the same motivation now that we had then. We wanted to be thin then and we want to stay slim now. The only difference is that, because we no longer feel the cravings and hunger that often went along with strong emotions (as well as at other times), we no longer experience an intense ''drive'' to eat. We may feel like eating sometimes, other than at mealtime, but it is easily managed. We have found out what it feels like to be nonaddicts.

We have found new and more appropriate ways to deal with our intense feelings. We have learned to *allow ourselves the right* to put a stop on the stress, speak out when we are angry, reach out when we're lonely, and rest when we are weary. We have learned that we have a right to nurture all parts of ourselves. We give ourselves permission to no longer be all things to all people. We want you to do the same.

## Stress, Anger, Loneliness, and Tiredness: Restoring Yourself in the Future

EXPERIENCE #10: FEEDING YOUR BODY: FEEDING YOUR SELF

Stress, anger, loneliness, tiredness. They confuse our bodies and our minds. They are hungers too, and if we don't satisfy them they will push us, often against our wills, to seek food.

The frustrations and angers, the moments of tiredness and isolation, will come again. It is essential that we give ourselves the peace of mind, open communication, companionship, and rest that will restore our bodies. Otherwise our bodies will seek false comfort in food.

Now it is time to let go of the stress, anger, loneliness, and tiredness that you have battled with in the past.

Tear all of the earlier Experiences out of this chapter and destroy them.

You may tear the Experiences into little pieces. Or you might want to burn them. We have had people flush them down the toilet or crush them up in a ball and stomp on them.

It may seem odd to destroy the Experiences that you have just completed. Most of us have been taught to respect books and to protect them. But you are more important than this book. Destroying the past and its hold on you is part of your breaking free. You will find that the most successful people in the world do not worship their past, but rather use it to gain important insights.

As you destroy each of the earlier Experiences in this chapter, close your eyes and return to your Circle of Success. Imagine it around you—encircling you, protecting you. This place of safety is the result of letting go of the past and the past's influence on your present.

You are safe and strong in your Circle of Success. Stand firmly and say *out loud:*

> "I am my own entrusted caretaker."

> "When my body is being pushed past its limits, I will speak up for myself and give it what it needs. When my mind is overwhelmed, I will speak up and demand the time or assistance that I require."

> "When I am angry, I will find a place where I can let go of my anger and the pain and frustration that lies beneath it. Whenever possible, I will state my feelings with simple dignity and honesty. I will give myself the care and respect I often demand that I give to others."

> "When I am lonely, I will seek the good company of people who value me. I will treat myself as I would treat a good friend."

> "When I am tired, I will give myself rest. I will allow my body and my mind the time and sleep it needs in order to renew itself."

> "In these ways and in others, I will nurture myself and care for myself, with love and with dignity."

> "Others may value me for what I can give, but I am more than this. I will appreciate me for what I feel, for what I

think, and for what I am. I am a living, human being. I deserve good and gentle care."

Now take this page and put it in your new Success folder or envelope.

Look at it regularly. Make sure that you are keeping your promises, taking the naps you need, getting the companionship and communication that you want and deserve. Most of us always have a few extra minutes for friends or family who need our help or our ear. But few of us will make the same time for ourselves. This is what we mean by a change in lifestyle. You would do it for others, so do it for yourself. Do it for life!

# CHAPTER 7

# Your Constantly Changing Body

The animal organism is subject to constant change. It is never quite the same for two moments.
—von Clausewitz

The only thing that remains constant in nature, is change.
—Prof. Richard F. Heller,
Opening Lecture, Mt. Sinai Medical School

## Bedlam Within Our Bodies

Our bodies are constantly changing. We change from minute to minute. We see something or taste something or even think of something and we are changed. Hormones spill into our blood, impulses race through our bodies, muscles contract, and blood vessels expand. Just as we are traveling at a rate of a thousand miles an hour on our rotating planet Earth and have no awareness of movement, our bodies are in constant flux, but we experience them as unchanging.

---

**Some changes are obvious; some changes are subtle. Some changes come easily and in predictable rhythms; other changes are less predictable and may signal "danger."**

---

Some changes are obvious: our faces flush or our legs cramp. Some changes are subtle: our pupils dilate to accommodate to a darkened room or our heartbeat slows as we move gently into sleep.

Some changes come easily and in predictable rhythms: the hormonal shifts that accompany menstrual cycles, or the changes in brain-wave patterns as we move through the phases of sleep.

Other changes are less predictable. They may come upon us unexpectedly. These changes may signal "danger," and we may experience them as jarring and, perhaps, frightening. The quick withdrawal we make when we touch a hot surface, for example, tells us that something nearby is capable of injuring us. The impulse to yell or to strike out in anger at someone may be caused by a similar evaluation that there is something hostile in the environment. In a moment our body's chemistry and our feelings, our reactions, are changed.

Multiply these momentary changes by a hundred and we have the variations that go along with pregnancy, changes in work, or sleep shifts. Multiply them by a thousand and we have the physical variations that come about with the grief of losing someone you love, the joy of the birth of a child, or the mixed emotions of your child's marriage. The body that used to smoke is not the same body that has given up the habit. The body you had at nine years old is not the body you had at sixteen, and the body you had at sixteen is not the body you have today. You are still changing, and as your body's chemistry changes, your thoughts and emotions change as well.

---

**The stars move across the heavens; the seasons come and go; our bodies change. Isn't it odd though that what we have come to expect in nature, we find so hard to accept in ourselves?**

---

It is amazing that with all this change, we are treated by others (and learn to treat ourselves) as if we were the same person that we were an hour ago, or a day ago, or even a year ago? Husbands and wives complain that their spouses are not the same person they married. Parents bemoan the fact that their sweet little baby has become a tormented and tormenting teenager. We complain that when we were younger we used to be able to eat anything we wanted without gaining a pound, but that now all we have to do is look at food and we gain weight. The stars move across the heavens; the seasons come and go; like everything in nature, our bodies change. Isn't it odd that what we have come to expect in nature, we find so hard to accept in ourselves?

## Medical Maneuvers

*Rachael:*

It was spring 1982, and I was recovering from brain surgery that had been performed only three days before. I was lying in my hospital bed suffering with what I estimated to be the worst headache known to mankind. While I knew, on some level, that every person coming out of brain surgery felt the same way, I was still pretty sure that my headache ranked up there with the best of them.

I was hot, sweaty, irritable. I buzzed for a nurse and waited for what seemed like a decade. She breezed into the room and inquired as to my "problem." I was hot, I explained, and asked that she turn on the fan. "Oh, now you're hot and need a fan," she complained. "Yesterday you were cold and needed blankets. Jeez! Can't you make up your mind?"

She flipped the fan switch and left me to my breeze and my thoughts. I felt angry and ashamed at the same time. I started to defend myself to an invisible judge. "It isn't me," I explained. "It's her problem, not mine. She was indignant because I happened to feel differently today than I did yesterday. In her mind, a day's passing should not have meant any change. To her I was the same person I had been twenty-four hours prior. She didn't consider that I could have developed an infection and a fever in that time or that the heating system might have kicked in or that some other unknown internal or external change could have occurred. As far as she was concerned, I was simply supposed to stay the same. "And," I concluded with a flourish, "she was indignant when I didn't act the way she wanted me to. Well—that was her problem, wasn't it?"

As I lay there thinking, feeling quite self-righteous over what I considered to be my unjust treatment, I knew that there had been times in the not-so-distant past when I had been just as demanding of other people. If friends changed plans, I accused them (usually without telling them) of being inconsiderate and fickle. If I saw a co-worker in the morning and was greeted warmly by her, I would be offended if I were ignored an hour or two later. When my boyfriend left me for my best friend, I vowed to make him pay for his betrayal. I treated myself and the world around me as if it were unchangeable; I even, I had to admit, based my deepest trust on the fact that my "good" friends could be counted on to think, feel, and act in predictable ways.

We're all like that. We expect others, and often ourselves, to remain the same, and we are upset when we see change. We demand consistency in a world of constant flux. The problem is that the world and everything in it does, in fact, change, and in many ways our happiness and peace of mind lies in our coming to accept change in others and in ourselves.

---

**At times, the medical establishment is no better than we are, unrealistically believing that in some ways we should remain the same.**

---

In many ways, the medical establishment is no better than we are, unrealistically believing that in some ways we should remain the same. It is customary policy in most hospitals, for instance, that upon admission each incoming patient must have a chest x-ray performed. If the incoming patient has a chest x-ray that has been taken within the last six months, the hospital says that the old x-ray is acceptable as a suitable substitute for a current x-ray. The assumption that these hospitals make is that the state of health of the patient's chest will not have changed over the past several months.

This hospital policy is clearly illogical. Pneumonia, emphysema, cancer, any number of diseases, can become obvious in a span of time less than a six-month period. The chest of the patient that was x-rayed fewer than six months ago is not necessarily the same chest that is entering the hospital now. Many changes may have occurred during that time. Yet hospitals ignore this obvious fact and continue to treat us as if we were unchanging. In other areas, the same hospitals are fully aware of the changeability of the human condition; for instance, they would never accept six-month-old blood tests or urinalyses. Still, in most hospitals, six-month-old x-rays continue to be accepted, and tradition, rather than logic, rules the day. The changeability of the human body is simply ignored.

Researchers are not necessarily any better at paying attention to differences or change than are physicians. Research findings that come from experiments involving young male subjects are used to make recommendations for middle-aged women. Even though age and gender can be very important differences, they are often disregarded.

We are all different, one from the other, but to make matters even more complicated, we ourselves change, from one day to another. Some physicians and researchers are beginning to pay attention to the ways in which these changes can affect our health. Recently, for example, scientists have found that timing cancer-related breast surgery at a certain point in a woman's menstrual cycle can greatly affect her chances of cure. This single medical issue is a hallmark for the attention that the medical community will soon pay to the impact of the body's changes on health and illness and recovery.

## Metabolic Turbulence

Nowhere is change more noticeable than in the area of metabolism—the ways in which our bodies break down and burn food. Here, change is constant. From minute to minute there are changes in blood sugar levels and insulin levels related to what we eat, what is stored as fat for fuel, and what is pulled out of storage for use. From hour to hour, normal daily rhythms guide changes in the amount of water we hold and the enzymes we release. Day to day and week to week, women's metabolisms are regularly affected by their menstrual cycle. The coming and goings of seasons, the regular changes in the length of daylight result in changes in us. Still, with the exception of premenstrual changes, which are finally being given some credence in the medical communities, we act as if our bodies are unchanging blocks of wood that do not, and should not, vary in any way.

"I don't know why I'm tired," we hear people say. "I really shouldn't be. I got plenty of sleep last night." "I don't know why I'm hungry," we tell ourselves. "I've had plenty to eat." "I don't know why I'm not losing weight as fast as I usually do," a friend will complain. "I'm watching what I eat." In each case the answer is the same. You are tired or you are hungry or you are not losing weight because you are a living being who changes from time to time. You cannot be expected to always respond like some machine that acts in the same way every time you turn it on.

Once we stop fighting change, we are better able to start understanding the changes that take place. In order to better understand what is happening *to* your body, first look at what is changing *within* your body.

## Hormonal Havoc

The changes that are related to your menstrual cycle or to pregnancy can cause havoc in the rest of your body. Increased cravings for starches or snack foods or sweets (or all three) can take you by surprise. If you are a carbohydrate addict, chances are premenstrual changes and pregnancy may be a chance to accumulate a great deal of weight and, wrongly, a lot of self-blame as well. The beginning of menstruation at puberty (menarche) and the end of menstruation in middle age (menopause) throw the body into a new kind of cycling, and can result in strong carbohydrate hunger.

---

**Carbohydrate addiction feels like the hunger and cravings you get right before your period—except, for the carbohydrate addict, it never goes away.**

---

Some nonaddicts find that right before their periods or during pregnancy, they become "temporary addicts." They suddenly take on the hunger and cravings and weight gain that most carbohydrate addicts endure most of the time. Although the physical changes that nonaddicts experience may not last forever, the weight gain and body changes that these episodes leave behind may last long after the body becomes "normal" again.

Many nonaddicts, who wouldn't normally understand the cravings that carbohydrate addicts typically experience, have greater sympathy when they are told that carbohydrate addiction "feels like the hunger and cravings you get right before your period—except, for the carbohydrate addict, it never goes away."

## Your Changing Body in the Past

### EXPERIENCE #11: ALMOST WITHOUT WARNING

We are so vulnerable. We know things will change but we hope, very hard, that they won't. When they do, we are almost always taken by surprise. Change is difficult for an adult. But the experience of change for a child or adolescent can be devastating.

Few parents are really able to prepare their children for change. Even though we hope that we have readied them, we know that they may not be ready for the shifts and transformations that they must face.

Dealing with external change is hard and stressful; when a friend moves away, we start a new school, or our parents divorce, we may silently endure our loss and feelings of insecurity. But when change takes place *within* our very bodies, the difficulties that we experience may be much, much more encompassing. They may strike us at our very core—we feel shaken, truly frightened, out of control. We may strike out or withdraw completely. We may put on a show or refuse to talk about our problems.

Think back to some of the times when your body was going through change. You might have been ill or frightened, you might have been reaching puberty, having a child, or approaching menopause.

Let your mind wander to your childhood and young adulthood, or even later, and finish each of the following sentences that are appropriate for you:

The first big change in my body that I was aware of was when I

_____

_____

_____

What did you feel? _____

_____

_____

What did you do? _____

_____

_____

At puberty, _____

_____

_____

What did you feel? _____

_____

_____

What did you do? _____

_____

_____

When I was pregnant (or thought I was pregnant), I _____

_____

_____

What did you feel? _____

_____

What did you do? _____

_____

_____

When I started reaching menopause, I _____

_____

_____

What did you feel? _____

_____

_____

What did you do? _____

_____

_____

When I have been sick, I _____

_____

_____

What did you feel? _____

_____

_____

What did you do? _____

_____

_____

When I have gained weight, I _____

_____

_____

What did you feel? _____

_____

_____

What did you do? _____

_____

_____

Let's look at your responses. If you are like most carbohydrate addicts, your responses to the last question, regarding weight gain, resulted in a more negative and self-blaming response than any of the others. Although weight gain may be no more your "fault" than puberty or illness, chances are you judged yourself more harshly in that arena than in any other. Although you may have asked for help when it came to other changes in your body, you probably did not seek out help when it came to understanding your weight gain. In addition, negative feelings about menopause, puberty, or debilitating illness may, in actuality, be the result of concerns about weight gain.

In this somewhat "enlightened age," most of us have been taught to accept and understand the physical changes that accompany puberty and aging. Yet most of us still feel ashamed and responsible for the changes that take place in our eating and our weight. We assume—and are told—we are to blame. We isolate ourselves and desperately seek quick solutions. We call ourselves names and base our happiness on one achievement—our ability to lose weight.

Learning to accept the changes that take place in our bodies, those related to weight-change as well as those related to age-change, is the first step in being able to take control of ourselves and our lives. Your weight reflects a great deal more than your ability to control yourself. It indicates how your particular body handles food energy, what signals it might be giving you, what needs it may be expressing.

You are more than a number on the readout of a bathroom scale. You are a complex organism and the sooner you stop blaming yourself and condemning yourself, the sooner you will be able to begin learning about this wonderful body that you have and, in the learning, be able to heal and help yourself to find true and lasting success.

## Your Changing Body in the Present

### EXPERIENCE #12: HOW DOES YOUR BODY RESPOND TO CHANGE?

Let's see how your body continues to be affected by change.

For each of the following situations that *apply to you,* circle the word that describes how your cravings for starches, snack foods, or sweets are affected:

Before my period, my cravings for starches, snack foods,
or sweets:                DECREASES     STAYS THE SAME     INCREASES

When I was pregnant, my cravings for starches, snack foods,
or sweets:                DECREASED     STAYED THE SAME     INCREASED

At change of life (menopause), my cravings for starches, snack
foods, or sweets:         DECREASED     STAYED THE SAME     INCREASED

In the summer, my cravings for starches, snack foods,
or sweets:                DECREASES     STAYS THE SAME     INCREASES

In the spring, my cravings for starches, snack foods,
or sweets:                DECREASES     STAYS THE SAME     INCREASES

In the fall, my cravings for starches, snack foods,
or sweets:                    DECREASES    STAYS THE SAME    INCREASES

In the winter, my cravings for starches, snack foods,
or sweets:                    DECREASES    STAYS THE SAME    INCREASES

When I am cooped up in the house or in the
office all day, my cravings for starches, snack foods,
or sweets:                    DECREASES    STAYS THE SAME    INCREASES

When I gave up smoking or chewing gum or some
other habit, my cravings for starches, snack foods,
or sweets:                    DECREASES    STAYS THE SAME    INCREASES

When I am happy, my cravings for starches, snack foods,
or sweets:                    DECREASES    STAYS THE SAME    INCREASES

When I am depressed, my cravings for starches, snack foods,
or sweets:                    DECREASES    STAYS THE SAME    INCREASES

When I am bored, my cravings for starches, snack foods,
or sweets:                    DECREASES    STAYS THE SAME    INCREASES

When I am worried, my cravings for starches, snack foods,
or sweets:                    DECREASES    STAYS THE SAME    INCREASES

After a worry has been lifted, my cravings for starches, snack foods,
or sweets is:                 DECREASED    STAYS THE SAME    INCREASED

When I have a cold, my cravings for starches, snack foods, or
sweets:                       DECREASES    STAYS THE SAME    INCREASES

When I feel irritable or out of sorts, my cravings for starches, snack
foods, or sweets:             DECREASES    STAYS THE SAME    INCREASES

When I hold in my feelings, my cravings for starches, snack foods,
or sweets:                    DECREASES    STAYS THE SAME    INCREASES

When I am doing something I don't want to do,
my cravings for starches, snack foods, or
sweets:                        DECREASES    STAYS THE SAME    INCREASES

When I eat certain foods, my cravings for starches, snack foods, or
sweets:                        DECREASES    STAYS THE SAME    INCREASES

When I get *less* sleep than usual, my cravings for starches, snack
foods, or sweets:              DECREASES    STAYS THE SAME    INCREASES

When I get *more* sleep than I'm used to, my cravings for starches,
snack foods, or sweets:        DECREASES    STAYS THE SAME    INCREASES

When I'm under pressure, my cravings for starches, snack foods, or
sweets:                        DECREASES    STAYS THE SAME    INCREASES

Sometimes, for what seems like no reason, my cravings for starches,
snack foods, or sweets:        DECREASES    STAYS THE SAME    INCREASES

When I have missed a meal or eaten
very lightly, my cravings for starches,
snack foods, or sweets:        DECREASES    STAYS THE SAME    INCREASES

**YOUR SCORE:**
Now let's see what your answers tell us about you and how your
body responds to change. Some of your responses may surprise you.
Count only the number of "decreases" and "increases" you circled
above (disregard the circles marked "stays the same").

Number of Decreases: _____        Number of Increases: _____

   **If you had an equal or greater number of "increases" than
"decreases" circled,** your body responds to change by pushing
you toward carbohydrate addiction. You may find that you can control your eating at times and then suddenly find the situation is completely out of hand. Your environment, your feelings, your body,
your thoughts, and your eating are all tied together. It is very difficult for you to control yourself over the long haul. You may start out
with a strong will and determination, but find that you seem to fade

over time. It is no wonder! Your body is very sensitive to the world within and around it. It is particularly crucial for you to learn to handle internal and external change in ways that will reduce your stress level. It is important for you to understand that your particular body is uniquely affected by change, and you must stop placing impossible demands upon it.

**If you had the same number of "increases" as "decreases" circled,** your body varies in its response to change. At times it may push you toward carbohydrate addiction, at other times it may not. Your hunger or cravings may seem to be under control for a while and then, suddenly, without reason you may find that your body seems to have a will of its own. What seems like the same situation may have no effect on you at times and then, at others, it may have an overwhelming impact. It is important for you to understand that change may have an unpredictable influence on you.

**If you had fewer "increases" than "decreases" circled,** your body does not seem to respond to change by pushing you toward carbohydrate addiction. Your hungers or cravings appear to be rather constant, and you seem to hold steadier than many of us. You appear to be able to separate your feelings from your environment, and you are less influenced by external or internal flux.

*Nina's Story:*

Nina B. calls herself a "Jekyll-and-Hyde Carbohydrate Addict." The substance that makes her into a "monster" is her monthly period. Three weeks a month, she is a steady, well-disciplined woman. She eats "healthy" foods and takes "pretty good care" of herself. But for six or seven days a month, a terrifying metamorphosis takes place. Influenced strongly by premenstrual fluctuations, she finds herself an uncontrollable "junk-food junkie" for about one week. She eats literally everything in sight: boxes of cookies, bread by the loaf with slabs of butter, pretzels, potato chips, ice cream by the pint, and "disgustingly sweet candy."

"I hate it. I work so hard on my eating all month," Nina has told us. "I watch myself like a hawk. I choose carefully, read labels, and give up a lot. Then all that work goes down the tubes. I find myself eating like a horse and gaining six or seven pounds in a matter of days. I hate my body. I hate myself."

Nina has told us that she dreams of having children (if she can find a decent guy) but fears that if she ever became pregnant "it would be nonstop eating for nine months. I'm even kind of glad there's nobody special in my life," she told us one day. "I would hate to have to make that decision right now."

Her family history supports her fears. Her mother, who also gained and lost weight in relation to premenstrual changes, gained 50 pounds with her first pregnancy and another 35 with her second. While carrying Nina, her mother developed gestational diabetes and was never able to take off the weight that she put on with the pregnancies. Her weight endangered her and her babies. Her cesarean delivery (second pregnancy) was complicated by her obesity, and her baby went home without her. Nina's maternal grandmother died shortly after childbirth, and although the information on the cause was limited, it seemed probable that a weight gain of about 60 to 70 pounds might have strongly contributed to it.

When Nina was given birth-control pills to regulate her period, she gained 20 pounds in five weeks, which she had never been able to take off. But more powerful than the discomfort she carries in relation to her weight is Nina's anger and blame of herself. This rules her thinking, her choices, and her life.

Though Nina's story is more extreme than most of the people with whom we have worked, the signs and symptoms of her metabolic mayhem are not unusual. Each of us is affected by our body's response to endocrine changes. Monthly cycles and pregnancy wreak havoc on some of us. Cramps, irritability, and bloating are not the only discomforts we may endure. Some of us may be spared one or more of these common problems, only to find that strong cravings for starches, snack foods, or sweets may accompany menstrual changes.

Long after the temporary fluctuations have subsided, the pounds may remain. And because we have come to think that we "should" be stronger than our bodies' impulses, along with the pounds comes a great deal of self-blame and shame. Ultimately, it is our fury and disappointment with ourselves that hurts us much more than the pounds themselves.

## Your Changing Body in the Future

### EXPERIENCE #13: DELIGHTING IN THE DISCOVERY

You already know a great deal about your own body and the ways in which it changes over time, but chances are you do not pay much attention to your needs. Instead of paying attention to our bodies' responses, we are taught to simply ignore them. Instead of loving and caring for ourselves, we are taught to demand that our bodies should not interfere with our work or our relationship demands. If we are tired, instead of taking a nap, we down another cup of coffee and push on. When the air is stale or the stress is too heavy and we end up with a headache, we pop a few aspirin and get back to the task at hand. Come to think of it, most of us don't even take the time to go to the bathroom until we can't "hold it in" anymore.

Even though we think we are getting away with giving them little attention, our bodies have ways of making their needs known. Too little sleep and too much coffee and you'll feel shaky or irritable or both. You'll take abuse when you needn't and become angry when you shouldn't. Too little fresh air and too much stress will run down your immune system and your supply of patience. Pretty soon, you'll get mad, go mad, or get sick.

On a daily basis, we push ourselves way past our natural limits and then wonder why we are tired and frustrated, and why, when all else fails, we simply burn out. Then we get a minimal amount of rest and start all over again. Deep within, we sense that we are hungry—hungry for sleep, hungry for rest, hungry for attention, hungry for appreciation, hungry for help, hungry for change. In an attempt to keep going a little bit longer we stuff food into our mouths, treating our bodies as if they were annoying children that we just want to quiet so that we can get on with our lives. But we *are* our bodies and this *is* our life. Sooner or later our bodies rebel. We start to forget things, become unwilling to do usual chores, become restless, bored, and simply lose all enthusiasm and motivation. Our weight will start to climb, and our self-image will plunge. We feel caught in some vicious cycle we barely understand.

When our bodies sense that there are unfulfilled needs, or during regular cycles, the endocrine system responds. Stresses, anger, frustration, and pressure all cause change within the endocrine system as we try to right the wrongs we do to ourselves. Normal fluctuations occur as well. Pressure headaches, irritability, loss of temper, even a feeling of hopelessness, may all be signs that your body is experiencing unfulfilled physical needs from internal or external demands. In the same way that pain is a signal that your body is in danger of being injured, feelings of depression or lack of clarity may be signals that your body is literally being pushed too far or too far at the wrong time. We may use food as a bribe to keep going until food itself also takes its toll and the whole system begins to fall apart.

Let us move on. Tear the first two Experiences out of this chapter and destroy them. Tear them into little pieces or burn them. It is important to let them go. You will get everything you need from your Future.

Return to your Circle of Success once again. Imagine that you are a living parent with yourself as your own child. As you stand in the center of your Circle, the child in you enters the Circle, and you open your arms to welcome and embrace the child.

This child is full of discoveries and excitement and, of course, full of demands as well. But you, as a loving parent (to yourself), will be patient and nurturing, helping the child to learn from his or her own experience. Mainly, your job is to listen, lovingly and caring, to the many changes that will mark this most wonder-filled journey of discovery.

Save this sheet for your new Success folder and place it inside after you read aloud these sentences. Come back and read them regularly. You may find that you see new things within them as time goes on.

"I will listen to myself . . . and to the changes that my body experiences."

"My body's voice may be quiet at first. It has been ignored many times and shamed as well. But soon, as it learns to trust me, it will grow stronger. A time will come when my body's needs will be expressed loudly and proudly and will not be ignored or hushed for any reason."

"I am not the same from day to day . . . or even minute to minute. I will not demand that I remain unchanged, but instead will welcome all the different aspects of myself."

"Like a rainbow of many colors, each beautiful and bright, my body flows from one state to another. Some days I may feel emotional, sensitive, and vulnerable. Other days I may be all work, ready to take on any task and unwilling to spend time on discussing feelings and such. I will understand that these changes and more are varied aspects of the wonderful organism that is me."

"I will not let other people try to push me into their way of acting or feeling. I will glory in the many faces of my body, my mind, and my feelings."

"Now is the time to stop: to stop the pushing, stop the demanding, stop the punishing, stop the pressure."

"I will take the time to listen—to the needs of my heart, my mind, and my body."

# PART III

# Your Mind: Your Will to Win

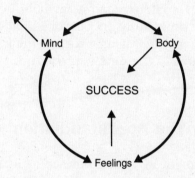

## A Mind of Your Own

Have you ever started off the day with every intention of staying on a diet, only to find that by the end of the day other demands have pulled you away from your goal? Do you find that your commitment to your diet fades as the day progresses, so that by evening your "will to win" couldn't care less? Have you ever told yourself that you will never succeed, that it's a hopeless cause, and that you had better get used to being fat or always hungry?

In each of these instances, you have experienced your *mind* pulling apart your Circle of Success. Your feelings may have tried to push you toward success with an irritability or a sense that things were "not right," feelings that wouldn't let you just eat in peace; your body may have contributed with a sinking feeling of disappointment, or both body and feelings might have remained silent—overpowered by your mind's logical (though erroneous) persuasion.

> **If you put your own needs before the needs
> of others in order to stay on your diet, you
> may be called "selfish" or "self-centered." If
> you don't put your own needs first, you will fail
> at your diet. Then they will say that you are
> "self-destructive" and have no willpower.**

When your mind pulls you away from your Circle of Success, you may wrongfully blame your body or your feelings. "I was so hungry," you say, "I couldn't stand it anymore," or "I guess I really didn't want to stay on it badly enough or I would have." But more often than not, you may be saying what you think *should* be the reasons you failed. Most of the time you may not really know.

## The No-Win Situation

You may be caught in what is known as a "no-win situation." That means that when you try to stick to your diet, you may find that no matter what happens—whether you fail or you succeed—someone, if only yourself, is going to be judging and blaming you. You lose either way. If you succeed, you will be blamed and criticized. If you fail, you will be blamed and criticized.

If, for instance, you sometimes have to put your own needs before the needs of others in order to stay on a diet, they may hint (or come right out and declare) that you are being "selfish" or "self-centered." They may not come right out and say it, but they will convey that message with a look or a tone or an attitude. They may even say that they want you to succeed, but their actions and manner tell you the opposite. If, on the other hand, you *don't* put your own needs first, you will fail at your diet. Then they will say that you are "self-destructive" and have no willpower. It seems as if you can't win either way.

> **If you do succeed in staying on your diet,
> your spouse complains that you're being
> "fanatical," your kids complain, and your
> friends feel offended.**

If you do succeed in staying on your diet, your spouse complains that you're being "fanatical," and says that you should be able to "relax once in a while," and breaking the rules "just this once" wouldn't kill you. Your kids complain that they want to eat *their* foods just like they used to and that they shouldn't have to "suffer" because "you're on a diet." Friends feel offended if you don't join them in celebrations, and family members feel hurt if you don't enjoy the foods they made "just for you." People put you in impossible situations, and given the demands, it's almost impossible to succeed. You find yourself filled with anger, resentment, or guilt. Your body wants to "give in." Your mind is pulled in many directions and can no longer help fight off the pressures that are tearing apart your Circle of Success. You may literally feel as if you are being torn apart.

The positive influence of your mind is essential to achieving your Circle of Success. The demands and criticisms of others (and ourselves) make success difficult to achieve and even more difficult to maintain. Even when you are able to harness the power of your mind to help you succeed, you may find yourself fighting to keep away the negative thoughts of yourself and others around you, pushing in on you and threatening your success.

> **Have you ever had the experience of saying
> something and realizing that you did not
> really mean it or even believe it?**

We are all susceptible to the influences of others. We may deny their words at first and then, almost without realizing it, we take in or "internalize" their thoughts. Have you ever had the experience of saying something and realizing that you did not really mean it or believe it? You may internalize the thought, even though it was not really "yours." In time, these thoughts can become part of us, setting up conflicts with the more essential, "real" us until we barely know who we are.

In the chapters that follow, we will explore, question, and sometimes challenge the thoughts and ideas that have come from your past, continue into your present, and may well influence your future. We will examine them, getting rid of those that interfere with your future success and strengthening those that will help insure your future joy and freedom.

# CHAPTER 8

# Your Will to Win,
# Your Will to Won't

He stands at war 'twixt will and will not.

—Shakespeare

## Accused, Tried, Convicted,
## and Sentenced—Without Proof

Imagine that you are walking into a restaurant and you notice a tall, slender woman sitting at the counter. She is eating a large hot-fudge sundae. You probably say to yourself, "Boy, does she have a great metabolism." If, on the other hand, you walked into the same restaurant and saw a short, stout woman eating the same sundae, you might think something like, "Boy, she wouldn't look like that if she didn't eat like that."

In the first case, we are assuming that the woman's weight is directly related to her metabolism—the way her body "burns" energy. In the second case, we assume the woman's weight is directly related to her eating—and to her ability to refrain from eating. We assume that the first woman's eating has no bearing on her weight but that the second woman's weight is all her "fault." If you continued thinking about it, you would probably come to the conclusion that the overweight woman had "no willpower" and that she "deserved" to be fat, even though she's not doing anything different than the thin woman is. The fat woman stands accused, tried, and convicted, and even sentenced to an undeserved fate by the mere fact that she's overweight. Not fair, is it?

This is an overriding prejudice in this country. It hides behind an assumption that is generally accepted as truth. The assumption is that overweight people have less willpower than slim people. This assumption has no scientific backing; it does not even go along with our own experience. Yet we still act as if it were, in fact, true. Now, we all know thin people who can't resist any "goodie" whatsoever and heavy people who have gone incredibly long periods with little or no food or who have stuck to virtually impossible diets. Still, the prejudice against the overweight is so strong that we tend to take as fact, and do not challenge, the idea that people who are overweight do not have enough "willpower."

---

**Although scientists have shown that people who struggle with their weight and with their eating have *no less* "willpower" than those who are naturally slim, the media and the medical community continue to blame us.**

---

Although scientists have confirmed that people who struggle with their weight and with their eating have *no less* "willpower" than those who are naturally slim and that in fact there is some evidence that we may have more, the media and the medical community continue to blame us for our inability to lose weight and to keep it off. The blame of others, though, would mean nothing if we didn't believe them and then come to doubt ourselves. Chances are, you already know that you can do many things when you set your mind to it. Still you have found over and over again that permanent weight loss has eluded you. It may have occurred to you that it doesn't make sense that you can do other things but not this one thing. If you have the willpower to put up with a crazy boss, or stick it out at night school, or refrain from killing your kids, how is it that you doubt that you have willpower? Why do you accept other people's proclamations about your ability to control yourself? Just because other people say it's so? Most of these same people fail in helping dieters 95 to 98 percent of the time. Why do you believe them?

We have *rarely* ever found a person with a lowered level of "willpower" in all the people with whom we have worked. The problem is that most of us have "won't power" as well as willpower, and the "won't" usually overpowers the "will."

---

**"Won't power" is made up of the fears, doubts, and unfulfilled hopes of your past experiences.**

---

"Won't power" is made up of the fears, doubts, and unfulfilled hopes of your past experiences. Your "won'ts" include the failures that you have yet to understand, the successes that you don't trust, and the influence of many people who often did not know what they were talking about. Your "won't power" came into existence long before you could separate the good advice from the bad, before you could question many of the rules and expectations.

The good news is that the "won't power" that breaks apart your Circle of Success can be eliminated, and we will help you do it. You learned your "won'ts" as a child, and you can unlearn them as an adult.

## Your Willpower/Your Won't Power in the Past

### EXPERIENCE #14: THE ONLY TASK THERE IS

Once upon a time, a student requested permission to study with a wise man. "Help me learn the wisdom of the ages," requested the boy.

"You have all the knowledge that you will ever need already within your own mind," answered the sage.

"But I thought so many thoughts. How do I know which are the wise ones and which are the foolish ones?" asked the boy.

"Ahhh," responded the wise man. "That is the only task to be undertaken."

Most of us are not used to paying attention to our own thinking or deciding which thoughts to trust and which thoughts *not* to pay attention to. The truth is that many of our thoughts date back to other people's influence. Some thoughts are helpful, some are not. Some thoughts are ours and some are not.

Not every thought that comes into our minds is one that we agree with or that we think is correct or valuable or right. Yet we often listen to our own thoughts without examining them. We do it by rote, without paying real attention to what we are saying or thinking . . . or doing. We draw conclusions that we know aren't exactly "right." We may even argue points that—deep inside—we know we don't believe in. Yet we argue them anyway, defending to the death our right to be—wrong.

These unexamined and often incorrect thoughts, doubts, sayings, beliefs can stand between us and our success. They are not, as they seem, unimportant points. They are rules for living and thinking that may hamper us in ways that we will discover in the pages to come. In many cases, these thoughts may prove to be responsible for some of your failures at dieting and perhaps other aspects of your life. They may lead you to trust other people more than yourself and to disregard important knowledge that only you have about you.

Think for a moment about the times that you have wanted to stay on your diet; you were motivated and able to handle yourself, you were sure of what you wanted and how to get it. Then a voice crept into your mind, a voice filled with doubt and criticism, a voice that tore apart the diet or your behavior or filled you with an insecurity that you didn't have before. You may have felt suddenly unmotivated. You may have had reasons to explain why the whole thing wasn't going to work anyway. That is the power of the "will to won't."

Complete the following sentences with the thoughts that come from your past:


I have trouble losing weight because _____

_____

_____

_____

When I go on a diet _____

_____

_____

_____

My cravings _____

_____

_____

_____

I love to eat _____

_____

_____

_____

For me, hunger and cravings _____

_____

_____

When I lose weight _____

_____

_____

_____

The food that I enjoy _____

_____

_____

The main reason my weight continues to be a problem _____

_____

_____

_____

    Now look over your responses. Do they come from your own experience or from what other people have told you about what _should_ be true, or are they some combination of both?

    For each question, ask yourself the following question: _Has this been my personal experience?_

    Most of us listen to others and to experts for so long that we forget which things we learned from our own experience and which things we were simply told by others. The beliefs that come from others may not be true for us and may eventually keep us from learning from our own experience. They help contribute to our "will to won't."

    Go back once again and with a pen cross out any of the sentences that are not truly _your_ sentences. You might simply cross them out or replace the words that you wrote with your own experience. No one need approve of what you wrote. You do not need to defend your thoughts. They are the result of your own experience and not the secondhand advice of others. It is time to leave behind other people's conclusions about their lives that they try to push on you. Each of us has enough work to do in life fighting our own negativity without fighting other people's negative thoughts as well.

## Your Willpower/Your Won't Power Today

EXPERIENCE #15: HOW STRONG IS YOUR "WON'T POWER"?

Let's see how strongly your "won't power" pulls at your Circle of Success. Dieters with a high level of "won't power" may use some of the sentences that follow to sabotage their own confidence in their dieting success.

Check off all of the following sentences that you have either thought to yourself or have said to someone else.

_____ "What makes you think this diet is going to work? You have failed every time before."

_____ "You're never going to do it. You might just as well get used to being fat."

_____ "They say it's unhealthy to go up and down in your weight, so you might as well stay at this weight and try to keep from gaining any more."

_____ "You can't go to someone's house and not eat what they serve because you're dieting."

_____ "It's okay to be on a diet, but other people shouldn't have to suffer because you're trying to lose weight."

_____ "If someone goes to that much trouble and makes something special for you, you can't hurt their feelings by refusing."

_____ "Don't be such a party-pooper. Just try to eat sensibly and go back on your diet in the morning."

_____ "A little will be okay. After all, it's your birthday!"

_____ "Relax and enjoy yourself. After all, you're on vacation."

_____ "You deserve it. You've been *so* good."

Count up the number of statements you checked.

**1–2:** Most of the time your willpower probably wins out over your "won't power." You are either very independent or very stubborn or both.

**3–5:** You often struggle to keep your own opinion in the face of what others say. Sometimes you win, sometimes you don't. Your willpower is strong but, even so, your thoughts can defeat you.

**6–8:** Your "won't power" interferes with your success much more than you would like. You start off strong and committed and then find yourself losing your "will to win." You sometimes think that you are your "own worst enemy."

**9–10:** You and others may have blamed you for not having enough willpower. You may be able to handle other parts of your life and not understand why control over your eating and your weight escapes you. You may be too concerned about other people's feelings. At times the needs of others may come in direct conflict with your own success. At these times, you may put yourself last.

The higher your score, the greater the sign that your "will to won't" is alive and active and may be overriding your willpower.

Your mind is an essential part of your Circle of Success. But often we are of "two minds"; part of us is pushing us toward success and part of us is pushing us away from success. When that happens, the result is a conflict within our Circle of Success and the circle breaks apart.

---

**You may not be used to questioning your own thoughts. Now we will listen to your thoughts, gently and with interest. Those thoughts that are worthy to stay will be treated with respect. Those thoughts that are not yours, those that you do not believe or want or respect, will be discarded.**

---

At first, you may not be used to questioning your own thoughts. You probably have simply accepted everything you thought as truth—your truth. Now we will listen to your thoughts, gently and with interest. Those thoughts that are worthy to stay will be treated with respect. Those thoughts that are not yours, those that you do not believe or want or respect, will be discarded. In this way your mind will be able to work in harmony with your body and feelings to guide you to the joy and freedom that is your right.

### Letisha's Story:

The first time we saw her, Letisha F.'s sweetness and shyness won us over completely. Her uncertainty was charming in its own way. Yet we knew that her apparent gentleness might stand in the way of her success.

"I've always been heavy," Letisha began, "and I've always blamed myself for it. But I've been following your program for nearly six months, and just like you said in the book, I'm losing weight, slowly and steadily. The cravings are almost completely gone but I still needed to see you because. . . ." She stopped. Tears filled her eyes and dropped to her folded hands below.

As her words poured out we heard a very familiar story. Letisha had grown up in a family full of love and caring, but also full of hidden demands. Letisha was supposed to be a responsible family member. She was given approval for what she could give to the family in terms of hard work around the house and contributed earnings as well.

---

**Although her family never spoke directly about her "weight problem," their actions implied that Letisha would not be as heavy if she did not "eat so much."**

---

Although her family never spoke directly about her "weight problem," their actions implied that Letisha would not be as heavy if she did not "eat so much." Letisha's younger sister tended to be much thinner by nature. Even though she ate as much as or more than Letisha, her weight remained lower. Still, Letisha's family gave smaller portions to Letisha than they did to her sister, implying that if she ate less, she would certainly weigh less. When Letisha complained about being hungry, her family would say, "You know we're only doing it for your own good," or "You know what will happen if we let you eat anything you want."

Pretty clothes were bought for her sister, and more practical clothes were purchased for Letisha. "After all," she was told, "you know how hard you are on clothes."

When work was required around the house, Letisha was called on to do it. If Letisha complained that she was doing far more than half the tasks around the house, she was reminded that she was the "bigger" of the two. "It was never that I was the older, but always that I was the bigger."

---

**Letisha was the "worker" in the family, valued for
what she could contribute, while her sister was
the "pretty one," valued for her attractiveness.**

---

Letisha received two messages from her family. The first was that she was the cause of the weight problem and the second was that she was the "worker" in the family, valued for what she could contribute, while her sister was the "pretty one," valued for her attractiveness.

Now, fifteen years older and 40 pounds lighter, these sentences were coming back to haunt her. While she was heavy she met and became engaged to a young man who valued her for her hard work and practicality. She had no need for "silly things, like so many other women," he would brag to his friends. She was happy wearing old clothes, didn't spend money on fancy hair stylists or makeup.

But Letisha's weight loss was challenging the role that Letisha's family had given her and that her boyfriend valued. Her "will to won't" was saying that a nice girl had no need "for such foolishness," but Letisha had other thoughts and desires. "A part of me says that I should be happy just losing weight and feeling good. But another part of me wants to make up for all the years I've lost. I want to spend all of the money I earn on clothes and makeup and . . . anything I want. It's my money and I've waited a long time to look this good. Other men are finding me attractive and it makes me feel . . . funny."

> **"A part of me says that I should be happy just losing weight. But another part of me wants to make up for all the years I've lost."**

"Another part of me says I wouldn't have to make up for those years if I hadn't made myself fat in the first place. I know you say that's not true, but I tell myself it anyway. Over and over. 'What does it matter how much weight you lost?' I say. 'What's the big deal? You wouldn't have had the problem in the first place if you weren't such a pig.' And then I feel ashamed. I don't know what to do. I don't know what to think." Her tears turned into sobs.

> **"Another part of me says I wouldn't have to make up for those years if I hadn't made myself fat in the first place."**

There, she had said it. She had let it out. Here was the crux of her pain. Although the thoughts that had been ruling Letisha's life were proving to be untrue, although her cravings were cut with a program that simply changed her body's biochemistry, although her parents' assumptions that her weight was her "fault" were no longer holding up, Letisha was still blaming herself for her lack of will-power and, of course, for her weight. Men other than her boyfriend were beginning to value Letisha; they said they appreciated her looks as well as her intelligence and not just what she could earn or do around the house. The truths that she had lived by were not being borne out by her experience.

The conflict that she was experiencing so deeply was tearing Letisha apart and threatening her continued success. Couples' counseling and lots of hard work led to a surprisingly happy result. Letisha learned to listen to her own experience and trust her own perceptions. Her new husband came to value all the new and wonderful aspects of Letisha, including her beautiful face and figure.

Letisha still finds it difficult to enjoy spending money and time on her appearance without the defending herself against her own negative thoughts and evaluations. But she forces herself to believe that she's worth it, and she says "I'm learning."

Many of us have stories similar to Letisha's. Some of us may not be as quiet or as humble as she, for we have learned to fight for what we want. But, like Letisha, we have been told by others the reason for our weight problems and what we should do about them.

All of us are affected by what other people tell us is truth. As children we are unable to close our minds to the negative influences around us. It is only as adults that we are free to choose which thoughts we will keep and which we will discard.

## Your Will to Win/Your Will to Won't in the Future

EXPERIENCE #16: TO EVERYTHING THERE IS A SEASON

You already know a great deal about your own thinking, but chances are you do not usually question the truth of your thoughts. Instead of questioning our own thoughts, we are taught simply to obey them. And rather than shedding our outgrown attitudes and values as we grow older and experience a wider variety of life, we are taught that to change our views is somehow disloyal.

We don't expect a teenager to be guided by the thinking of a four-year-old; if we did, that adolescent would never cross streets or venture out into the world. Yet we expect a fifty-year-old to be guided by many of the same thoughts that we learned thirty years prior. But years ago we were different, and so was the world.

It is time for change, change in thinking that comes from challenging what we may have taken for granted and which now must bear the weight of close scrutiny and examination. We cannot expect to change our lives unless we change our thinking as well. Even the Bible says that "to everything there is a season and a time to every purpose under heaven." The thoughts of our youth are no longer right for us. Let us challenge them and, if we find them wanting, let them go.

Tear the first two Experiences out of this chapter and destroy them. Tear them into little pieces or burn them. Let them disappear. They are sentences, thoughts, and opinions that are no longer valid or important in your life.

From this chapter, tear out the sheets that follow. Carry them with you for a week and fill in your thoughts, one day at a time. If, after a week, you wish to continue, make up new sheets for yourself. Save the sheets and place them in your Success folder.

For each day of the week, fill in thoughts about your weight, your eating, or dieting that come to mind. After you write down each thought, look at the sentence and decide whether or not *you* think that it's true. Do not be persuaded by what you have always been taught is true or what "everyone knows" is true. The only truths that we are concerned with here are *your* truths.

If you think that the thought that you have just written down is true, leave it. If you think that it is no longer true or, perhaps, was never true, cross it out. Once a thought has been crossed out, do not reread it. If you are unsure as to whether or not you think the thought is true, put a question mark before it and leave it.

In the days to come, take these sheets out again. You may add additional pages if you like. If some time has passed, read over the sentences that are not crossed out. If you find that they are no longer true for you, cross them out. Remember that life is change. Your body changes, your feelings change, and in the same way, the thoughts within your mind will change as well.

**Day 1**   Date _____

1. _____

   _____

2. _____

   _____

3. _____

   _____

4. _____

   _____

5. _____

_____


**Day 2**  Date _____

1. _____

_____

2. _____

_____

3. _____

_____

4. _____

_____

5. _____

_____


**Day 3**  Date _____

1. _____

_____

2. _____

_____

3. _____

_____

4. _____

_____

5. _____

_____

**Day 4**  Date _____

1. _____

_____

2. _____

_____

3. _____

_____

4. _____

_____

5. _____

_____

**Day 5**  Date _____

1. _____

_____

2. _____

_____

3. _____

_____

4. _____

_____

5. _____

_____

**Day 6**  Date _____

1. _____

_____

2. _____

_____

3. _____

_____

4. _____

_____

5. _____

_____

**Day 7**  Date _____

1. _____

_____

2. _____

_____

3. _____

_____

4. _____

_____

5. _____

_____

# CHAPTER 9

# The Levels of Addiction

**Addict** From the Latin *addictus,* given over; one awarded to another as a slave.

—*American Heritage Dictionary*

## Standing on the Edge of Quicksand

Do you find that trying to stay on commercial weight-loss programs and diets usually becomes harder as time goes on? Does the desire to cheat, which you may control relatively easily at first, become more difficult to handle each time it returns? As the cravings get stronger, does your resolution to follow the diet "exactly" become weaker?

We hear it from almost every carbohydrate addict who comes to see us. "As time goes on, I can feel myself getting closer and closer to 'giving in.' Pretty soon, I know it's only a matter of time. Eventually I come up with some excuse that gives me permission to eat the foods that I wanted all along. But it's not the excuse that's important; it's the growing, nagging desire to let go."

*Sondra's Story:*

Sondra H. was only twenty-two when she first came to see us, but she had already been on "at least seven or eight diets—maybe more." She was finishing up her college education, graduating with a degree in fashion design.

147

---

**"I need some help. I've been fighting this all of
my life, but before it was just about boys and
clothes. Now, it could mean my whole career."**

---

"I need some help. I've been fighting this all of my life, but before it was just about boys and clothes. Now, it could mean my whole career. I'm the fattest student in the whole school. Fashion is our lives. I even started making my own clothes because I couldn't find anything decent to wear in my size.

"What finally got me to come to see you was one of my teachers. They had this career planning seminar at school—you know, for graduating seniors. She didn't mean to be cruel, she was really trying to help, but in front of all the students, she suggested that maybe I could go into fashion design for 'big women.' I thought I would die. And the worst part of it was that all the kids were sitting around a table—including this guy that I've had a crush on for two years—and they all nodded and agreed that that was a great idea! I couldn't believe it!

"I've been on every diet in the world. They all start out the same," she continued. "I'm really gung-ho at first. I tell myself that this time I will do it, and for a while I follow the diet perfectly. I eat all the right foods. It's easy because I generally like a lot of foods. I enjoy salad and vegetables and fruit. It doesn't look like I am going to have any problem that I can't handle. At first, I don't eat any candy or anything. I grab a piece of fruit or something instead of junk and I'm okay."

---

**"I suddenly know that I'm going to cheat. It
may not be right away, but sooner or later . . .
I don't know *how* I know, I just know."**

---

"Then, without warning, I suddenly know that I'm going to cheat. It may not be right away, but sooner or later . . . I don't know *how* I know, I just know. I start craving everything in the world. I don't have any desire for good food anymore. It's like suddenly I'm out of control and I try to convince myself to hold on, but I know that sooner or later I'm going to lose it.

"It's like standing on the edge of quicksand. You just wait there, on the edge. Maybe you call for help or maybe you've learned that no one can really help you anyway. And you just stand there, telling yourself that this time you'll keep it from happening but knowing that sooner or later you are going to take the first step and then . . . it's all over.

"It has happened enough times for me to know exactly what to expect, but that doesn't make any difference. I'm powerless to stop it. No matter how hard I try—I mean, I can swear that this time will be different—I still end up taking the first step and even if I try to climb out again, and even if I succeed for a time, pretty soon I'm sinking to the bottom of the pit.

"I don't know what you can do. I don't know what anyone can do, but you helped my sister so I thought maybe . . . you could. The truth is, I don't know what else to do."

## The Levels of Addiction

Sondra did not know it but she had already given us all the information we needed to start to help her. In describing her problem, she had mentioned all three of the illusions that are telltale signs of a carbohydrate addict's thinking.

Each of the three Levels of Addiction contains a key illusion. This illusion guides your thinking and influences the choices that you make. Each new illusion replaces the illusion that has come before. With each new illusion, the carbohydrate addict progresses to the next level of thinking, feeling, and hunger that will eventually lead to loss of control and, for many of us, leads to our own destruction.

Loss of control does not happen "all of a sudden." It might *feel* as if it comes on without warning, but it follows progressive levels that can be predicted and, best of all, can be halted. Once you have learned to identify your level of thinking, you will be better able to turn and walk away from your own personal pool of quicksand.

## LEVEL #1: The Illusion of Denial

### *The Illusion:*
At the first level, the illusion is denial: you believe that you don't "really" have a problem. This thought often comes to mind at the

very beginning of the diet or even as you are choosing a diet to follow.

At this level, you will probably tell yourself that dieting is "just a matter of willpower" and that you "can do it if you really want to." Gone from your memory are all the times that you have said the same thing to yourself only to find yourself unable to follow your own advice later.

If you do think of past failures at this level, you attribute them to one of two things: you probably say that you didn't succeed at other times because of a lack of motivation or because of something or someone that was pulling you away from your goal. In either case, you assure yourself that this time is "different," that you really won't have any problem.

At Level 1, most people tell themselves that they "just love to eat," but this illusion hides the fact that they have a progressive disorder that mimics a nonaddict's love of food *only in the beginning*. At this level, if others mention past failures, most carbohydrate addicts chalk the comments up to jealousy or to the fact that they "just don't understand." At *later* levels, your desire for food will make it obvious that there is something different in the way you respond to food as compared with other people, but by the time that you come to this realization, your eating or your weight may well be out of control.

### The Feeling:

At the first level, denial can lead you to feel pretty confident; that is what is so sly and seductive about this illusion. Because you are busy denying that you have any problem at all, you may experience a false sense of security that can spread to other aspects of your life as well.

When you are in the throes of this illusion, you feel better than you have for a long time. Family members, friends, or co-workers may remark on your good humor. In the back of your mind, you may have some slight misgivings but you shrug them off and, in general, you feel ready to take on the world. Self-assuredness, tinged with tiny moments of doubt, mark the feeling of this level.

### The Hunger:

At this level, you enjoy a wide variety of foods: vegetables, salads, meat, fish, poultry, or dairy foods are combined with breads, pastas, fruits, and desserts. Your meals are balanced because you enjoy the diversity. Your preference for many foods reinforces the false belief that you do not have an eating problem and that you will be "just fine" on this diet.

## LEVEL #2: The Illusion of Control

### *The Illusion:*

At the second level the illusion is that of control: you believe that your hunger and cravings are manageable through willpower. In some cases, it becomes a matter of principle; you are determined to get "a handle on this thing." At this level some people voice the same thoughts and advice that others have told them in the past, but to which they refused to listen. Now, in a sort of desperation, they try hard to make themselves believe that "it's just a matter of control."

At this level, you will probably find that you judge yourself by your ability to control your eating and, therefore, by your weight. When you are able to stick to your diet, you feel great. You tell yourself that you are terrific. "See," you say to yourself, "all you needed to do was use a little willpower." On the other hand, when you "cheat" or break your program, you may be merciless and unforgiving.

At the second level, some carbohydrate addicts try to go it alone, while others seek professional help. In either case, however, most people repeat the same basic attempts at weight loss that failed them in the past.

### *The Feeling:*

When carbohydrate addicts first enter Level 2, they may think that they are sure of their ability to control themselves, but their feelings may show that they have some doubt. After they have been at Level 2 for a while, carbohydrate addicts feel noticeably less confident. As they begin to see that their addiction is more than just a matter of self-control, the illusion starts to break down. Most carbohydrate addicts admit to feeling disquieted or irritable and some say that, as the control slips away, they experience a feeling of panic.

### The Hunger:

At this level, you will experience an increasing desire for carbohydrate-rich foods like breads and pasta, potatoes, rice, fruits, and fruit juices. Sandwiches become more attractive than platters. Snack foods (potato chips, pretzels, popcorn, cheese puffs, and crackers) may become a more frequent treat. You may have less of a desire for vegetables and salads, either choosing them less frequently or taking smaller portions of them in comparison to bigger servings of bread, pasta, or pizza.

## LEVEL #3: The Illusion of Defeat

### The Illusion:

At the third level, the illusion is of defeat: you believe that you are doomed to failure and that no one can help you. You may consider giving up completely. You convince yourself that you have tried everything and nothing works. You may blame yourself or the medical community or your genes or your family (or all of the above). You have no patience with listening to a friend's enthusiastic story about how this newest diet worked for "someone who was heavier than *you!*"

You tell yourself that it's hopeless and that you had better just get used to it. You are concerned about your health but don't really think there's much you can do about it. You may avoid seeing your physician. You probably avoid social occasions as much as possible. Family gatherings become just another chance for people to judge you, and you're already doing enough of that for everyone.

If you had been trying to lose weight by dieting alone or with the help of a professional, you eventually give up all attempts to stick to the program. You have a harder time consistently staying with your exercise or activity regimen. In order to feel better, you may tell yourself that you will stick to certain "sensible" guidelines, but you never actually spell them out in detail or follow them.

### The Feeling:

The Illusion of Defeat can lead to powerful and devastating feelings. You may feel almost powerless to express your feelings. You may feel ashamed or trapped or overwhelmed. All of the good that you have done in life may seem insignificant compared to the fact that you cannot control your eating and your weight. You feel as if everyone is judging you, and when they do, they see you as less than adequate.

Carbohydrate addicts at Level 3 often go back and forth between feelings of hopelessness and anxiety. They may feel as if they should be doing something but don't know what to do. Level 3 addicts may express the feeling that they have "given up," but they rarely feel the peace of resignation. In the beginning they may feel discouraged, but later they often say that they barely feel anything at all.

Some carbohydrate addicts tell us that they "really don't care anymore." This seems to be a kind of defense mechanism that lasts for only a short time. Underneath their indifference is a desperate cry for help.

### The Hunger:

At this level, continual snacking takes the place of separate and distinct mealtimes. A desire for sweets (candy, cake, cookies, ice cream, donuts, chocolate, and puddings) increases. You will continue to experience a desire for starches, such as breads and pasta, potatoes and rice, but you will find that you have much less interest in meat, fish, poultry, salad, and vegetables. Some Level 3 carbohydrate addicts enjoy fruit and fruit juices, whereas others have no desire for them at all. Snack foods will probably remain a regular treat. Sandwiches are probably your only form of "meal"; you rarely sit down and eat a full, well-balanced dinner unless you are invited out.

The *way* in which you consume your food will often change in Level 3. Most food is eaten out of the container or drunk out of the bottle. Rarely is the table set for meals unless other people are present.

*True* Level 3 carbohydrate addicts, who are deep into their addiction, may find that at times they don't even enjoy eating. They may eat just because they "have to." As the cravings increase, Level 3 carbohydrate addicts eat whenever they can and whatever they can. They can no longer deny, even to themselves, that their eating is completely out of control.

## Levels of Addiction in Your Past

EXPERIENCE #17: YOUR PERSONAL ADDICTION PROFILE

Every carbohydrate addict has a personal profile that chronicles his or her movements through the levels of addiction. Some carbohydrate addicts move quickly from one level to the next. Some move easily from Level 1 to Level 2 and remain there, and never going on to Level 3. Some carbohydrate addicts move up and down the levels in response to menstrual changes, stress, or dieting demands.

Let's take a look at your Addiction Profile. It will help us to understand *your* particular patterns of movement through the addiction levels.

Fill in the spaces below that seem appropriate to you.

If a sentence doesn't seem to apply to you, leave the space blank and go on to the next sentence.

If you are filling in a blank and a certain instance comes to mind, use it.

If no one example comes to mind, take your answers from your general past experience with food and dieting.

Don't worry if you find yourself mixing and matching responses related to more than one diet. Most of our patterns remain the same no matter which program we're attempting to follow.

In the past, before I would begin a diet "officially," I would eat

_____

and I would feel _____.

Sometimes I would think _____

_____

When I first began a new diet I would eat _____

_____.

That would make me feel _____

_____.

and I would begin to think _____

_____.

Within _____ hours/days/weeks/months I would notice

a change in my _____.

My mind was saying _____

but _____.

The biggest change was in my _____.

_____

For instance, _____

_____.

One of the most important patterns in my thinking is _____

_____

_____

One way that I fool myself is that I _____

_____

_____.

If I were going to help someone else diet successfully, I would __

_____

_____

_____.

In addition, I would _____

_____

_____

_____

Look at your answers to the Addiction Profile. You probably know a great deal more about your own eating patterns than anyone else who has told you how to control your eating and weight.

Read over your last two pieces of advice. Can you use them yourself? If not, why not? If so, take time to write down the details carefully. Put these suggestions in your Success folder for use when _you're_ ready to use them.

## Your Current Level of Addiction

### EXPERIENCE #18: WHAT IS YOUR LEVEL OF ADDICTION?

Write the word _yes_ or _no_ in response to each of the following sentences. Write _yes_ if you generally agree, _no_ if you do not agree.

Some of the sentences that follow may seem to be similar to others, whereas some sentences may seem to say contradictory things. Respond to each sentence as if it stands alone. Do not worry about being consistent.

YES OR NO

_____  (1)  I just _love_ to eat. I enjoy foods of all kinds.

_____  (3)  I don't like to admit it, but I often eat large portions of my meals out of the can or box.

_____ (2) I've been eating mostly meat-and-potatoes kinds of foods, basically protein and starches, and not many salads or vegetables.

_____ (1) Lately I've been enjoying a wide variety of foods, especially vegetables and salad.

_____ (3) I'm getting to the point where I just don't care.

_____ (3) My family's eating patterns have set me up to be fat for life.

_____ (1) *What* you eat is an important part of keeping your weight under control. It's very rare to see a fat person who eats healthy food.

_____ (2) I wonder why I am successful in other things in my life, but I am still not able to control my eating and my weight.

_____ (1) A good basic rule of thumb is to eat low-calorie, low-fat food, and to eat until you feel satisfied. That will pretty much keep you slim for life.

_____ (3) I eat most of my meals "on the run."

_____ (1) I think that most people could control their eating if they just ate less of everything.

_____ (2) Lately I've been more and more concerned about my eating and my weight, although I would certainly not say I was "very worried" about it.

_____ (2) I snack a little, but I balance it with regular meals.

_____ (1) Sometimes, in the back of my mind, I wonder if I'll be able to take off the weight for good, but in general I feel pretty confident.

_____ (2) I tend to eat more starches and snack foods than vegetables, but I don't eat too many sweets.

_____ (3) I often fall into a "drugged" sleep after eating.

_____ (3) I wish I would just give up and stop fighting this "losing battle."

_____ (2)  I could live on bread and butter.

_____ (1)  I enjoy breads and pasta and such, but not much more than the average person.

_____ (2)  I am pretty sure that I could control my eating if I _really_ wanted to.

_____ (1)  I enjoy a piece of fruit for a snack or for dessert.

_____ (3)  I've been feeling trapped by my own eating, but I've tried everything and nothing works.

_____ (3)  I think that I might be one of those people whose fate it is to be fat.

_____ (1)  A little moderation in food, as in all things, is the answer to most weight problems.

_____ (2)  I find that I'm often tired in the afternoon or right after dinner.

_____ (3)  If I'm alone, I don't take the time to prepare "real" meals.

_____ (3)  Sometimes I eat even though I'm not really enjoying the food.

_____ (2)  Weight control is like many other things; it simply takes discipline.

_____ (1)  My meals are made up of a balance of proteins, vegetables (including salads), and carbohydrates. I don't eat more of one type of food than another.

_____ (2)  I had been feeling pretty much like I had my eating under control, but lately it's been slipping.

**SCORING YOUR LEVEL OF ADDICTION QUIZ:**

Circle your "yes" answers only.

Count up your number of "yes" (1) answers and place in the space below.

Count up the number of "yes" (2) answers and "yes" (3) answers and place these numbers in the appropriate spaces.

Number of "yes" (1) answers _____
Number of "yes" (2) answers _____
Number of "yes" (3) answers _____

Let's look at your answers. The group in which you have the greatest number of answers indicates your current level of addiction. If you have the same number of answers in more than one group, you probably move back and forth from one level to another.

Example: Julia's answers looked like this:

Number of "yes" (1) answers ____4____
Number of "yes" (2) answers ____8____
Number of "yes" (3) answers ____7____

Julia's answers indicate that she is largely at Level 2. But the number of "yes" answers she has in Level 3 are very close to those in Level 2. At times of stress or when she is premenstrual or simply as she grows older, Julia will probably find that she moves into Level 3 more and more frequently.

Your score indicates your own personal level of addiction, but your level can change from day to day or, in some cases, from moment to moment (though most of us stay at one level for a while). The feelings and hungers that we feel are often a combination of many levels, but the illusions that we associate with our own particular level of addiction tell us a great deal about our thinking in relation to our weight, our eating, and ourselves.

## Your Levels of Addiction in the Future

### EXPERIENCE #19: A LEVEL BEYOND

Carbohydrate addiction is real. But although your cravings may be driven by a physical force within you, your mind can trick you into thinking that you aren't addicted or that you can control yourself. You may tell yourself that nothing can help. All of these are example of the illusions that influence your mind as you progress through the levels of addiction. All of them are untrue.

You have completed the first two Experiences in this chapter.

Now it is time to let go of the illusions that keep you trapped in your addiction and tear apart your Circle of Success.

Tear the first two Experiences out of the chapter and destroy them. You may tear the Experiences into little pieces or burn them. Get rid of them forever. If you think that you need to look back at them or hold onto them, that is just another illusion. It is time to let go of the past.

You do not need to look to your past and remember old illusions. We will help you to recognize and challenge any future illusions that arise.

Take the chart that follows and put it in your Success folder. Look it over at regular intervals, perhaps once a week.

Note, on the back of the chart, the date and the level of addiction at which you seem to be. In the days between your self-evaluations, pay attention to the thoughts and behaviors that mark that level. The simple act of being aware of what you are doing and what you are thinking will often stop your progression to higher levels or bring you to lower levels of the addictive process.

Freeing yourself of the addiction process altogether—being on none of the levels—often means being aware that you *are* addicted, that your thoughts and hungers and feelings push you to lose control and that there are things that can be done to help you to gain and maintain control. It means knowing that you are free to choose the foods that you want to eat and learning to handle the physical part as well as the psychological and emotional parts of your addiction. Ultimately it means healing your mind, your body, and your feelings so that no part of you is in conflict with any other part.

Use the chart that follows to identify and challenge your thoughts and to recognize the feelings and hunger that mark the different levels. Write down your thoughts and help yourself to be free of the pain and illusion of the past. When you are finished writing and ridding yourself of your old pain and old thinking, destroy the past (and the paper) and move on to a new and free tomorrow.

## LEVELS OF CARBOHYDRATE ADDICTION

| Level | Hunger | Thoughts & Feelings |
|---|---|---|
| #1<br><br>The Illusion of Denial | Desire for foods of all kinds:<br><br>Salads<br>Vegetables<br>Fruit and fruit juices<br>Beef<br>Lamb<br>Pork<br>Chicken<br>Cheeses<br><br>At Addiction Level 1, "good wholesome meals" are desired and enjoyed. | At Level 1, the carbohydrate addict often has the illusion that there is no problem. Carbo addicts may still experience a false sense of security. There are often some mild concerns about weight, which are calmed by rationalizing that the food that is being eaten is "healthy" and that "good food never hurt anyone." There is a lack of awareness that this is the first stage of a progressive disorder. |
| #2<br><br>The Illusion of Control | An increasing desire for carbohydrates in the form of:<br><br>Breads, rolls, bagels<br>Potatoes<br>Rice and rice cakes<br>Pasta, spaghetti<br>Snack foods of all kinds<br>   potato chips, popcorn, pretzels,<br>   cheese puffs<br><br>Less desire for vegetables and salad.<br>There *may* be some desire for beer and wine. | At first, the carbohydrate addict may believe that he or she is still "in control" of eating, but later there is concern over eating and weight. There may have been several attempts to lose weight with some success at first, followed by a regaining of lost weight. There may be tiredness around 2 to 3 P.M., as well as some tiredness after dinner. In the evening, there may be a desire for snack foods. |
| #3<br><br>The Illusion of Defeat | An increasing desire for sweets as well as snack foods:<br><br>Breads, rolls, bagels<br>Cakes, candy, cookies<br>Chocolate<br>Pies and puddings<br>Potato chips, popcorn, pretzels,<br>   cheese puffs<br>Rice, potatoes, pasta<br>Sandwiches of all kinds<br><br>Snacking and sandwiches take place of regular meals. | At this level, eating may be less pleasurable and more of a compulsion. There may be great concerns about weight and control of eating. Several attempts at dieting, in the past, may have failed. This level is marked by tiredness and self-blame. There may be a sense of being trapped or feeling overwhelmed. The carbohydrate addict may isolate him- or herself, feeling a desire to "just be left alone." |

# CHAPTER 10

# Your Internal Judge

He who judges himself, condemns himself.
—H. G. Bohn

*Joan's Story:*

Joan L. was an intelligent and pleasant woman. A clinical psychologist by profession, her training was just more "proof" to her that she was a failure:

"I hate it. Here I am, a trained professional and still I am fat, for all the world to see. It's affecting my personal life and I'm starting to think it's having an effect on my practice as well.

"I'm divorced and I'll be fifty-two next week. My personal life goes up and down with my weight. I use the personal columns to meet new people. Sometimes I answer ads, sometimes I put in ads of my own. Do you know how many men put 'Wanted: slim woman' into their ads?"

---

**"My weight can vary by fifty or sixty pounds. I have four sizes of clothes in my closet. Closets, I should say. I have a 'fat' closet and a 'thin' closet."**

---

"My weight can vary by fifty or sixty pounds. I have four sizes of clothes in my closet. Closets, I should say. I have a 'fat' closet and a 'thin' closet. I even put a mirror on my fat closet for a while, so that I would punish myself when I went to get dressed in the morn-

**163**

ing. Then I thought that I should be putting the mirror on my thin closet to reward myself for losing weight. It's a moot point now. While I was moving it, it broke and I threw the #!**! thing away.

"When I'm at a high weight, I tell myself that if I will just take off some weight, I will answer any ad I want. I promise myself that I will put in ads of my own that will sound more confident and even a bit sexy. I figure that if I look good, I will let myself sound it and show it. But as my weight goes down, my thinking changes. I tell myself that I will look 'silly' if I act like this or that I really 'shouldn't' dress like that.

"When I'm at a high weight, what I do and what I say are always under scrutiny. I'm always judging myself. It's as if I'm never good enough. I never leave myself alone.

"You would think that it would change when I lose weight, but even when I succeed and slim down a bit—for a while—it's still not good enough. 'Look at your skin,' I say to myself. 'You wouldn't have those stretch marks if you hadn't been so fat.' Or if I buy something nice to wear, I tell myself 'You look ridiculous in that outfit. Everyone will laugh at you behind your back. Who are you trying to fool? You look like a pig.' "

---

**"Losing weight is important to me.
But I want to be happy as well."**

---

"Losing weight is important to me, that's why I'm here. But I want to be happy as well. I keep thinking that my weight is the key, but I don't know anymore. I just feel like I'm never good enough, though I know that I'm a nice person, a good person. When I do something well, I praise myself a little, but when I do something wrong, I never let myself forget it. Somehow it's tied up with my weight and somehow it's got a life of its own.

"The irony is that I'm a psychologist. I am supposed to help other people to get what they want in life, but I can't even help myself."

# When Good Is Not Good Enough

*Richard:*

There is an epidemic that, day by day, is spreading through this country. It is ruining the lives of people who might otherwise be happy. It gives them no peace of mind and far less satisfaction. It affects their relationships with their friends, spouses, and children. It can make work a nightmare. This is the disease we call "perfectionism."

---

**While they may be somewhat understanding when it comes to others, perfectionists are unforgiving slave drivers when it comes to themselves.**

---

Men and women who might otherwise be considered rational and sane become obsessed with achieving and maintaining a level of perfection that is pretty much unreachable. While they may be somewhat understanding when it comes to others, perfectionists are unforgiving slave drivers when it comes to themselves. They rarely realize how demanding they are of themselves and how their perfectionism is ruining their chances for happiness and success. And the tension that they experience affects those around them.

When it comes to weight loss and dieting, perfectionism runs rampant. A person who has 5 or 10 pounds to lose becomes haunted by his "excess weight." A healthy young woman carrying the extra pounds gained during pregnancy looks for a place to lay the blame in every part of her mind and soul. A mature woman, who should have the right to enjoy a well-earned retirement, is so unhappy with her eating and her weight that she can find no peace of mind.

I am certainly *not* recommending that no one lose weight or that we shouldn't want to lose weight. I am *not* saying that we should no longer look for the cause of the weight problems that confront us. I have devoted my life to helping people correct their eating and weight difficulties.

What I *am* saying is that we should have reasonable, realistic goals for ourselves; goals that can be met, and in meeting them, allow us to feel *good* about our success.

It has been my experience that women are far harder on themselves than are men in all areas. I am not sure if women tend to be more perfectionistic because they so often find themselves in positions where they are being judged by others or because they have to be "extra good" in order to succeed in this society. In any case, men are less likely to condemn themselves for a less-than-perfect job, whereas woman regularly accuse, try, and execute themselves.

---

**"I *should* be able to lose five pounds the first week. I must be doing something wrong" or "There's no reason why I shouldn't have lost more weight than that. I'll just have to eat less" are statements that we are far more likely to hear from women than from men.**

---

## A Matter of Sex

In the area of weight loss and eating control, particularly, women are *far* more demanding of themselves than are men. "I *should* be able to lose five pounds the first week. I must be doing something wrong" or "There's no reason why I shouldn't have lost more weight than that. I'll just have to eat less" are statements that we are far more likely to hear from women than from men. That doesn't mean that men are less concerned with losing weight or less motivated, just that they don't seem to be quite as demanding of or as angry with themselves.

Perfectionism is an excellent example of the mind pulling apart the Circle of Success. The greater the demands we place on ourselves in terms of doing things "the way they *should* be done," the less likely we are to get them done in the first place.

### *Rachael:*

I have struggled with perfectionism all of my life. Though I love to communicate, my fear of not being perfect used to make writing lectures, articles, papers, even letters, a virtual nightmare. Even while I was working on something that I knew didn't have to be perfect, a voice in me would not let me rest.

Even as I wrote, I told myself that people wouldn't understand what I was saying unless I was much more specific. I would slave over everything that I produced, rewriting it time and time again. When I wrote letters, I imagined that the recipients would think poorly of me if I wrote in a phrase by hand that had been left out when I was typing. By the time I finished worrying about it, it was easier to type the whole letter out again. I would watch time slipping away but something in me kept pushing me to do it "right."

---

**When it comes to dieting and weight loss, perfectionism is an almost certain way to bring about failure. Isn't it ironic that by trying to do something very well, we keep ourselves from being able to do it at all?**

---

When it comes to dieting and weight loss, perfectionism is an almost certain way to bring about failure. Isn't it ironic that by trying to do something very well, we keep ourselves from being able to do it at all?

## When the Body Rules

When you are perfectionistic about losing weight, you have rules in your mind that may have nothing to do with your body's reality. When you decide what should happen when you lose weight, you use guidelines that come from your past, from others, or from parts unknown. You apply other people's experiences to your body and expect your body to meet your demands.

For instance, have you ever decided how much you "should" lose within the first week of your diet? That expectation probably came from your experience with what worked for you at other times, perhaps when you were younger. Or it might have been based on how much weight a friend lost. Have you ever figured, based on a certain weekly weight-loss average, how much you "should" weigh by a certain date? Have you ever concluded that you weren't losing weight "fast enough"?

These expectations come from the assumption that your body is like a machine and that if you give it so much to eat, it will always give you so much weight loss. Well, as we know, when it comes to losing weight our bodies don't work like that. The body rules. It can be guided and influenced by what you do but, in the end, your body is going to do what it is going to do—and you have only a limited amount of control over what will happen.

---

**Your body can be guided and influenced by what you do, but in the end, your body is going to do what it is going to do—and you have only a limited amount of control over what will happen.**

---

The same thing happens in relation to dieting. You may think that you "should" be satisfied with a certain amount of food or that you "should" be able to stick to a given diet but, the truth is, your body may have a different opinion. And that opinion is the one that counts.

Expectations about dieting and weight loss are important; they can help us plan and change our lives. When our expectations are not met, however, most of us blame ourselves for not meeting our own demands. We are so hard on ourselves, in fact, that we make it less likely that we will learn from our own errors and, in many cases, less likely to try again. And when we judge ourselves harshly, we become frightened of our own thoughts and then, even when we do succeed, we don't enjoy the success that we have earned.

Carbohydrate addicts are particularly prone to perfectionism. In many cases, they have been judged by other people all of their lives. If you are heavy and you are eating what any normal-weight person eats, someone is sure to comment on your breaking your diet. If you stick to typical diet foods, someone is certain to ask you about your diet and about how much weight you have lost. If you lose weight, people remark how much "better you look." If you gain weight, you are open to being teased or shamed. Some folks even have the audacity to tell you that they are being cruel "for your own good."

---

**At every social occasion, we are open to criticism
about what we are "doing to ourselves."**

---

At every social occasion, we are open to criticism about the amount and the kinds of food we eat and what we are "doing to ourselves." Is it any wonder that we end up judging and blaming ourselves and finding ourselves lacking?

## The Judge That Comes from Your Past

EXPERIENCE #20: THE CRIME . . .

Recall a time when you wanted to do something right and, for one reason or another, you failed. Perhaps you did not really fail, you simply might not have done as well as you would have liked. Or you might have done well but someone else had higher expectations of you. Perhaps you didn't get the grade in school that you wanted, or something you were making didn't come out perfectly; perhaps you lost something. It happens to all of us. But for some of us, such events can leave permanent scars.

Close your eyes and remember where you were and what was happening.

What happened? _____

_____

_____

How old were you then? _____

_____

_____

Where were you? _____

_____

_____

What were you doing? _____

_____

_____

What were others saying? (Try to hear their actual words). _____

_____

_____

_____

What were you thinking? _____

_____

_____

What did you say? _____

_____

_____

What would you have liked to say that you held back? To whom

would you have said it? _____

_____

_____

Now close your eyes again and let yourself, once again, experience what you were feeling. Let the feelings and memory come through. Don't hold your feelings back. Write down what you remember feeling.

_____

_____

_____

_____

That experience may still be influencing the decisions you make and the ways in which you view and judge yourself. We'll take a closer look at them in the next Experience.


**EXPERIENCE #21: . . . AND THE PUNISHMENT**

We often make decisions or judgments about what to do in the future based on the kinds of experiences we looked at in the last exercise. Let's go back to that experience now using our minds rather than our feelings.

Write down the judgments that you made *about yourself* from that experience or from any other past experience.

Example:

If you had been planning to buy someone a birthday gift and you lost the money, you might write something like: *I learned that I am careless and that I cannot be trusted with money.*

If there had been a time when you wanted to do well on a test but you got very nervous and didn't get a good grade, you might write something like: *I realized that I'm not as smart as I think I am* or *I learned that I don't do well under pressure.*

Now think back to your past. Remember the times that you "failed" to do as well as you or someone expected. The events might be from your childhood or it might have been not so long ago. Below, briefly describe the incidents and list the judgments you made *about yourself at the time.*

1. _____

_____

_____

_____

2. _____

_____

_____

_____

3. _____

_____

_____

_____

4. _____

_____

_____

_____

5. _____

_____

_____

_____

6. _____

_____

_____

_____

If you need more room, take the time to write down the rest of your thoughts on another piece of paper.

These are important incidents and the judgments that come out of them can help shape the way you see yourself and judge yourself for the rest of your life. Your success in dieting and in many other aspects of your life can literally depend on your ability to challenge and remove these judgments from your mind.

## The Judge That Still Remains

### EXPERIENCE #22: ARE YOU A PERFECTIONIST?

We are not used to listening to ourselves—that is, to the comments that we make when we are "thinking out loud" or to the little "unimportant" things we say to other people. Although we may be taken aback when we hear the words of our parents come out of our mouths when we speak to our children or to other people, in general, our thoughts come and go and we pay them little attention.

Sometimes what we say is important because it shows us the thinking that is going on right below the surface. This is especially true when it comes to the judgments we make about ourselves and the expectations we have for ourselves. Let's look at the expectations that you carry with you today and see if perfectionism is pushing apart your Circle of Success.

Check off (✓) any off the following sentences that you agree with. If you notice that you have an emotional response to a statement—if you feel like crying, if you feel upset, annoyed, or angry—then put a double check (✓✓) in front of the sentence.

If you have "always hated" a particular saying, that is reason enough for a double check (✓✓).

If a sentence is one that you don't agree with, leave the space blank (___).

____ 1. Only the best succeed.

____ 2. Sometimes good just isn't good enough.

____ 3. When you succeed they rarely remember, when you fail they never forget.

____ 4. That which does not kill you makes you strong.

____ 5. Never take "no" for an answer.

____ 6. One flawless performance is worth a dozen mediocre attempts.

____ 7. Second best is not good enough.

____ 8. Winners never quit and quitters never win.

____ 9. To give your all, totally and without thought, is success.

____ 10. That which you have failed at is only that which you have not devoted yourself to.

**SCORING THE JUDGE WITHIN:**

Count up the checks you made; count a double check as two.

**1–2:** You don't seem to be very judgmental or perfectionistic. Or you have worked very hard at learning to appreciate and accept yourself. In any case, perfectionistic thoughts do not seem to present an obstacle to your future success.

**3–5:** There is a struggle between the part of you that is easygoing and the part of you that demands perfection. You may find that you blame yourself either way. If you do things with little concern, you feel guilty. If you spend a great deal of time on a task, you blame yourself for the wasted energy. You need to learn to let go of the thoughts that judge you and cause you pain.

**6–8:** You tend to be very hard on yourself, but your "saner self" tries to talk reason. You never feel comfortable doing less than your best and so you dislike being rushed. You don't feel comfortable until you are sure that your work is acceptable. Your perfectionistic thoughts cause you mental and perhaps physical unease.

**9–10: (or above)** You have a very hard time letting yourself do anything less than your best. You may try to not be hard on others, but you are very demanding of yourself. You take on too many tasks because you believe that no one can do them as well as you. You get upset when time pressures and lack of cooperation make you hand in a "second-rate" job. You get frustrated with people who don't seem to care about their work. You know that you are hard on yourself, although you have to admit, it's an attribute of which you are proud.

The higher your score, the greater your perfectionism. It is important to do things well, but how well they should be done should be based on the demands of the job rather than the demands of our self. If we constantly judge ourselves and find ourselves lacking, or if we must perform incredible feats in order to appease ourselves, our mind is most certainly pulling apart our Circle of Success.

## Banishing the Judge from Your Future

### EXPERIENCE #23: THE ONLY PERFECTION THERE IS

The Internal Judge. He sits within our mind and makes judgments as to whether we are good enough or slim enough, whether we try hard enough or are nice enough. He never lets us rest. We keep trying to please a voice that is, after all, within us.

A mind that is driven by perfectionistic demands cannot find rest or satisfaction or freedom or happiness. The more demanding our judge the more difficult it is to achieve success. Our decisions are clouded by fear of our own disapproval. We make choices that are based on avoiding blame. We are often tired and worried and our personal and professional relationships suffer.

The closer we come to understanding how to achieve success, the more we realize that perfectionism has no place in our lives. We want to do well, to accomplish a great deal. But we want to make wise choices as well. And most important of all, we want to enjoy all that we have worked so hard to attain.

Now is the time to redefine perfection. Rather than the striving for some unreachable pinnacle of exactness, let us define perfection as allowing ourselves to be all that we can be—right now. Perfection is the expression of our talents, the enjoyment of our abilities, the pleasure of the job, and the joy of the moment.

It is time to let go of the frustration, stress, anger, and distress that come from continually judging ourselves.

Tear the earlier Experiences out of this chapter and destroy them. They are no longer relevant to your success. You may tear the pages into little pieces; you might want to burn them. You can crunch them, stomp on them, or pour dishwashing detergent on them. Get rid of them. They are gone.

Now close your eyes and enter your Circle of Success. This is a place of safety for you in which no one judges you or finds you lacking.

Say the following sentences *out loud:*

"I am perfect just the way I am."

"I am good and kind and *I* like me. I do not have to prove myself to me or to any other person."

"When I have a job to do, I will trust myself to put the amount of work and energy into it that seems appropriate. I do not have to do a flawless job. The perfect job is that which is called for at that time."

"I am more than the number of pounds I weigh or the size of clothing that I wear. I will not judge myself by my weight."

"I will try to eat in the way that I think will bring me good health and happiness. I will not choose a diet that is inappropriate because I think that I 'should' be able to meet any eating restriction or dietary demand."

"If I am unable to stay on my diet, I will gently examine what led to the difficulty. I will not blame myself. I will make sure that I am not expecting too much of myself, and if I find that this is the case, I will get the help I need to make it more likely that I will succeed in the future. I will not blame myself nor place impossible demands on myself."

"If others attempt to influence me or judge me, I will ignore their words, understanding that they place similar demands and judgments on themselves."

"In these ways and others, I will become a good and trusted friend, a forgiving companion, to my self."

Now take this Experience and put it in your Success folder.

Look at it regularly. It is easy to slip back into perfectionistic and judgmental ways. Others will try to make demands on you. They will tempt you with the reward of approval or threaten you with their disfavor. Do not be swayed.

No one's approval amounts to anything compared with your own liking of yourself. Stay strong and stay focused.

# PART IV

# YOUR FEELINGS: THE INTERNAL TIDE

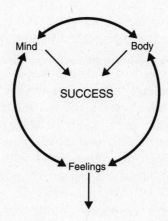

## The Rise and the Fall

Have you ever experienced a sudden and complete loss of motivation? There you were, going along fine, on your diet, and poof, suddenly, you had no desire to keep going. You weren't aware of any event that had happened or any thought that in particular upset you, you simply found that you no longer cared or felt involved.

Have you seen a stubbornness in you, bordering on rebellion, creep into your thoughts? Is there a part of you that declares mutiny on your diet and says, "Hey, I've had enough of being 'good.' It's time for some fun"? And, with that, does your work or your diet get put on hold?

That was your *feelings* pulling apart your Circle of Success.

**181**

When your feelings pull you away from your Circle of Success, you may wrongfully blame your mind or your body. You may, for instance, attribute a dieting "slipup" to your hunger or your cravings. But there's an easy way to tell the difference. Stop for a moment and think about what went on inside you right before the "slip." Were you really experiencing a craving for the food? Or, rather, did you just feel that you "didn't care"? If you didn't care, that was a prime example of your feelings pulling apart your Circle of Success.

## Who's the Boss?

Most of us think that our feelings don't have much impact on our actions. We think that we are guided largely by our thinking. But that's not true. Our feelings influence us in every aspect of our living and, in many cases, we twist and turn our thinking so that it ends up supporting our feelings, rather than vice versa.

How many times have you wanted to eat something that was not allowed? Your thoughts were saying "No! No!" but your feelings were saying "Yes! Yes! Yes!" Guess which won? Not your thoughts. Generally, your feelings put a great pressure on your thoughts and thought often gives in. This is a perfect chance to see conflict and harmony in action.

If you wanted to eat the goodie in question but were unable to convince your thoughts that this deviation from your diet was okay, chances are that you ate it anyway and felt a bit uncomfortable. Or, if you didn't eat it, you felt deprived. Both are examples of two of the essential parts of your Circle of Success in conflict. If, on the other hand, your mind gave in and agreed that "this little piece wouldn't hurt you" or that you could afford a "splurge," you probably enjoyed the treat—a fine example of harmony. Later, however, your mind probably regained its composure, and once again, conflict returned.

Do not underestimate the power of your feelings. They can convince your mind that it is wrong, and they can change the very biochemistry of your body.

It is only by directing your feelings toward success that you can keep your Circle of Success intact and working for you. Many people will tell you to disregard your feelings or to put them aside for the moment. Don't be fooled. Your feelings are very powerful and, one way or another, they will have their way.

In working with other professionals, we often hear them boast as to how they performed this operation or gave that lecture even though their own lives were falling apart. The true mark of a professional, they will tell us, is the ability to separate feelings from the demands of the job. We have found that this is not so. We would state rather that the true mark of a fool is one who thinks that they can do it.

Your feelings will not be ignored. Face them, deal with them, respect them, and satisfy them. Bargain and compromise, if you must. But in any case, do not turn your back and walk away from them. They will not be disregarded, and sooner or later, you will find that your feelings have influenced parts of your thinking and your life in ways you never anticipated.

Feelings are not your enemy. Rather, they are your friend. They are you. Just as pain in your stomach warns you that something is harming you, painful feelings tell you that danger is present.

In extreme cases you may marshal your inner resources and coerce your thoughts into overpowering your feelings. Feelings may protest over and over again, but thoughts use the power of logic and may resort to name-calling, enlisting the support of embarrassment and shame. Feelings learn that their messages are unimportant. They become quiet and soon they are silenced.

Now we feel nothing. We may have thought that this was the way out of conflict, but emotional numbness is not the way to harmony. With feelings silent, we can feel no joy, and no true freedom or success can ever be attained.

Your feelings are an essential part of your Circle of Success. They must be respected and understood. They are the messengers of joy as well as pain. They are powerful friends and must be respected as foes. They can work for or against your Success in infinite ways.

Most of us spend a great deal of time listening to other people's feelings, but don't take the time we need to listen to our own. Your needs, your desires, your sensations, and your hopes are a wonderful gift. Enjoy them and learn from them. They are vital to your Success.

# CHAPTER 11

# Going Strong ... Then Going, Going, Gone

My strength shall be made perfect from my failures.
—New Testament

We have all been through it. You're doing well on your diet. You're "on a roll." You have no intention of cheating. Your weight is coming down and you feel good. Then, for what seems to be no reason, the whole thing falls apart.

It may happen at a party or a family gathering; most likely it happens when you are all alone. You know you shouldn't be eating it. You may not even want it. You feel deprived, or angry, or tired or rebellious or . . . you just are sick of being told what to do.

You may tell yourself that "this little bit won't hurt" or that you'll go back on the diet in the morning. And maybe you will. But before long you are off the diet more than you are on, and within a short time, other demands for your time and attention take over. The weight comes back, and although you may feel like you failed, there's a part of you that doesn't really care.

What is happening here? Why do people who seem to be doing well experience this kind of "motivation slippage"? Why do we cheat on diets? Do we feel guilty or just feel like we *should* feel guilty? What can you do when you don't want to do anything?

# Diet Slip-ups in the Past

### EXPERIENCE #24: KNOWING WHOM TO LISTEN TO

*Rachael:*

There is a song that I used to love about twenty years ago. I think it was called "Second Story Window" (though I never did know why). The words described how hard it was to know who your friends are. That's how I have often felt about my own thoughts and feelings as well. Sometimes I'll feel very strongly about something; it will feel as if it is the *real* me speaking. I will defend it to the death. Then, two days later, I can't imagine how I could ever have felt that way.

When it comes to dieting, we see the same thing. Thoughts and feelings can be our best friends or our worst enemies. The trick, as they say, is to know who your friends are. The song says that you can tell "by lookin' in their eyes"—and that's exactly what we are about to do.

In the Experience that follows, you will be asked to write down both your feelings and your thoughts. Although we talk about feelings and thoughts as if they are separate in this Experience, in real life things, we know, are not so clear-cut. You may have thoughts about your feelings and feelings about your thoughts.

For now, consider thoughts to be the sentences that cross your mind; those phrases that you could express to others. Thoughts might include: "You can't stay on a diet all your life. You have to have fun sometime," or "Forget about the diet. Just eat healthy things in sensible amounts and you'll be just fine."

List the following as feelings, sensations, and emotions that have single words to describe them like: hot, angry, cold, disappointed, afraid, angry, stressed, proud.

Now, think about your past diet experiences and complete the sentences that follow. Fill in as many thoughts or feelings that you can remember.

*Very important:* This is not an exercise about blame. We are simply trying to understand how your thoughts and feelings affect your success in dieting. *For once in your life, put your blame on hold.*

Remember to include as many details as possible when you complete these sentences:

*Successes*

In the past, some of the *thoughts* that have helped me to resist temptation were: _____

_____

_____

_____

Some of the *feelings* that helped me to successfully resist temptation have been: _____

_____

_____

_____

When I do well on my diet I *think:* _____

_____

_____

_____

When I do well on my diet I *feel:* _____

_____

_____

_____

*Slip-ups*

In the past, some of the *thoughts* that have crossed my mind right before I broke my diet were: _____

_____

_____

_____

Immediately before breaking my diet I have *felt:* _____

_____

_____

_____

When I *don't* do well on my diet I *think:* _____

_____

_____

_____

When I *don't* do well on my diet I *feel:* _____

_____

_____

_____

Now, let's look over your answers and see what they tell us about you.

Count up the number of "think" answers and the number of "feeling" answers you had in the preceding Experience. Each answer within a sentence counts as an separate thought or feeling. If you filled in three thoughts or three feelings for a single statement, that counts as 3.

Count your answers up and list them separately under "Success" and "Slip-ups" below:

*Success*
Number of Feelings _____ Number of Thoughts _____

*Slip-ups*
Number of Feelings _____ Number of Thoughts _____

Your answers give us an important clue as to whether your feelings or your thoughts (mind) help you to stay on your diet or push you to break it.

If you had a greater number of feelings than thoughts under Success, you can probably be sure that your emotions can be counted on to support you in your dieting success. If you had more thoughts, your mind is a strong and reliable friend. If the numbers were just about equal, your mind and feelings work well together in keeping your Circle of Success in harmony.

If you had a greater number of feelings than thoughts under Slip-ups, your emotions can get in the way of your success. If you had more thoughts, your mind is a strong opponent. If the numbers were just about equal, your mind and emotions can at times combine to cause conflict in your Circle of Success.

## Diet Slip-ups in the Present

### EXPERIENCE #25: A TEST OF EMOTIONS

Let's take a look at how emotional a person you are. Certainly our feelings change from day to day and sometimes from moment to moment. Different people can bring out the emotional side of us. So can stress or concerns about time or money. Still, it all evens out in the end. Check off all of the following emotions that you think you generally experience in a given week.

If your feelings intensify right before your period, take the test twice. Let one set of answers reflect how you feel for the week right before your period. The other set of answers will tell us how you feel "in general."

During most given weeks, I feel the following emotions at least once:

| | | |
|---|---|---|
| ___ joy | ___ envy | ___ anger |
| ___ affection | ___ compassion | ___ sadness |
| ___ hate | ___ excitement | ___ fear |
| ___ love | ___ pride | ___ embarrassment |
| ___ zeal | ___ worry | ___ sorrow |
| ___ sympathy | ___ happiness | ___ irritability |
| ___ fondness | ___ freedom | ___ passion |
| ___ shame | ___ warmth | ___ nastiness |
| ___ rebelliousness | ___ mischievousness | ___ jealousy |
| ___ indifference | ___ revengefulness | ___ willfulness |

**SCORING YOUR EMOTIONAL LEVEL:**

Most people label feelings as "positive" or "negative," but in this chapter we are interested in learning about the strength of your feelings and their impact on your mind and body.

Count up your checks and read over your score. Remember that premenstrual changes, stress, and feelings of loss can temporarily change the strength of your emotions.

**SCORING THE EMOTIONS:**

**0–10:** Your answers indicate that your feelings do not usually overpower your thinking. When you make up your mind, you are probably able to stick to your plans. Be careful to give your feelings a chance to express themselves in positive, constructive ways so that you can keep your Circle of Success in harmony.

**11–20:** You may often find your thoughts and your feelings in conflict. You sometimes get angry at yourself for being so emotional. One part of you may be saying one thing and another may be pulling you in a different direction. You may find yourself influenced by the people around you. Conflict between your mind and feelings may often pull apart your Circle of Success.

**21–30:** You are strongly influenced by your emotions. You feel things deeply and may not always be able to express all that you experience. People who are guided by their thinking do not understand you. While it is important to honor all of the positive power within you, be sure to be guided by good judgment in order to keep solid your Circle of Success.

## EXPERIENCE #26: THE COLORS OF LIFE

You are more than the sum total of your body, your mind, and your feelings. You are the unique way in which the essential parts of you act, react, interact, and intermingle. Someone once said that your body gives you limits, your mind gives you direction, but your feelings give you life. The emotions that you hold within you are powerful and real. They cry out to be heard. There are few friends who can routinely handle sharing our feelings. There are few of us who are easily able to handle our own.

The process of understanding, owning, respecting, and honoring our own emotions is important to our success. When feelings have no place to go, when they are denied, shamed, and hidden, they will pop up in unexpected places. Like an angry child who has been denied his or her moment in the sun, feelings denied will tear at whatever is near.

Have you ever had a feeling of love that was denied? Your body turns cold. The feeling hides and turns and changes. Resentment grows. Old angers and shame come to the surface. Feelings do not just fade at someone else's command. They come back, twice as strong, but changed in the kind of emotion they carry.

Let's explore the power of your feelings and discover where they live in your body.

Choose a back and a front picture that represents your body from the pages that follow. For this exercise you will need a box of crayons or colored pencils that have at least 30 colors. Do not use colored markers; you will need to be able to make the color deeper or lighter depending on the intensity of the feeling.

Look at the first emotion in the three columns in Experience 25. Choose a color crayon that represents that emotion to you. On the front and/or on the back of the picture, find a place where you have felt that emotion. Color in as much of the area(s) that seem to represent the feeling. Bear down harder or color a wide area to show that you feel the emotion intensely. When you have finished coloring in that area(s), put that color aside.

Do the same with all of the emotions listed in Experience 25. If you do not feel any particular emotion in your body, let it go and move on to the next feeling.

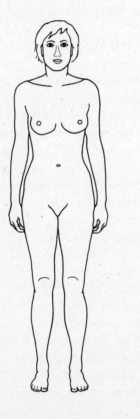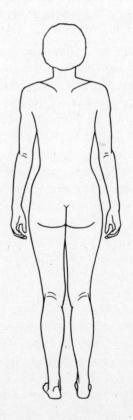

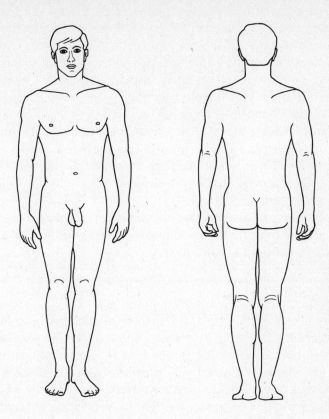

When you have finished filling in the pages, look at your pictures with a loving and caring eye.

The emotions that you have experienced are important; they are vital to your success. One by one they have communicated with you; they have allowed you to experience them and know them. If we do not understand and honor our feelings and give them a place in the Circle, they will most certainly lead to conflict.

Now, find a comfortable place to sit. Close your eyes and allow yourself to concentrate on each part of your body and the feelings that reside there. Breathe deeply and slowly. Start with the top of your head and move gently down the front and back of your body. With each feeling, stop and take in long, slow breaths. Then, let them out. If memories come to mind, do not stop them. Let them in and experience them. If you feel like crying, let it out. These feelings are part of you.

When you have moved through each part of your body, continue to breathe deeply, and if you like, allow yourself to fall asleep.

When you wake, write down the feelings and thoughts that came to mind as you traveled through your body and, perhaps, through your dreams.

Without looking at your picture again, destroy it. Destroy your answers to the earlier Experiences in this chapter as well. You have already moved on in your life. These were the feelings of the past, feelings that followed you into the present but will not follow you into your tomorrow.

As you destroy each of this chapter's past Experiences, feel the cool breeze of the promise of tomorrow cross your face and remind you that, in letting go, you are free.

## *Doris's Story:*

Doris T. was thirty years old. This was the first time she had been to the Carbohydrate Addict's Center. She told us that she had been "a bit chunky" all of her life but had *really* put weight on with her second pregnancy. "When I was pregnant with my first daughter I was sick as a dog. I couldn't eat anything. Sometimes I could barely keep water down. The doctor thought he was going to have to take me into the hospital and feed me intravenously. He said it was the first time that he ever saw morning sickness last nine and a half months. I left the hospital weighing 16 pounds less than I did before I became pregnant.

"With my second daughter, it was as if I made up for the first pregnancy and another two to boot. I swear I started craving food from the moment of conception. I simply could not get enough to eat. I went to the same doctor and I thought he was going to go crazy. With every visit it looked like I went up another notch on his scale. He started to make me come in more often. He was afraid of a diabetic pregnancy; I was afraid I was going to burst. This time, I left the hospital weighing 73 pounds more than I did before I became pregnant.

"It's been almost three years and I'd like to try for a little boy, but my doctor says that he doesn't want me to even *think* of it unless I can take off at least 50 pounds. The problem is that I'm getting older and I can't just sit around and wait until some of the pounds come off. I've tried a couple of diets, liquid fasts, even diet pills for a total weight gain of about 10 pounds.

"In the next couple of years I'm going to have to make some kind of a decision. Also, if I'm not going to get pregnant, I want to go back to work. We can use the money and I can't keep putting my life on hold waiting to see if I can lose weight."

Doris decided to give losing weight one more try and came to the Center. After spending two weeks learning about the program, she began the diet. For the first six weeks, she felt "fantastic." Her cravings were gone and she had no difficulty in sticking to the guidelines. She lost weight each week and was feeling very good.

On her seventh week, Doris showed no weight loss; her eighth week showed a gain of about half a pound. In the past, Doris would have given up. "I know myself. That happens every time. I'm fine as long as the weight is coming off, but when I hit a plateau it's all over. It doesn't matter that I know it's childish. I just lose all motivation."

But this time was different for Doris. Armed with an understanding of which feelings came right before her diet slips, Doris made a plan. While she was still experiencing the weight loss of previous weeks and her feelings of excitement with her new diet were still strong, she wrote letters to herself to be opened "in case of emergency." She numbered the notes and put them away.

As her weight loss slowed and her motivation began to slip, Doris pulled out the letters she had written to herself and opened one each day. There, in her own writing, were words of encouragement that reminded her of her purpose and gave her renewed strength. She stayed on her diet, and after two more weeks of staying the same weight, she began to lose weight once again.

"I never could have done it if I didn't know my own patterns. I thought all of those diets that I failed at before were just a waste of time and energy, but now I realized that I learned something from them all. This time I didn't let my own feelings get me down. And I never will again."

## A Future Free of Diet Slip-ups

EXPERIENCE #27: LOVE LETTERS

Now it's time to write yourself the words of encouragement that you may need to help you in your journey to success.

Think of the advice that you have given so caringly to others. Now you have a chance to offer yourself the kind of friendship that you have wanted to give and to receive the caring that you truly deserve.

Carry these sheets with you and when a "message to yourself" crosses your mind, write it down. Don't put it off. These will be the best love letters you may ever receive. For one week, write yourself a loving letter of encouragement every day.

The letters may all be different or they may have the same theme. Make them positive and helpful. Include the advice that you would give to other people. Even if you don't have the courage to follow your own advice now, include it in the letter. Tell yourself how you feel and what you want to see happen in your life. Be open, loving, honest.

When you have finished a letter do not read it over. Your emotions do not have to get approval from your mind. Quickly fold up the note and put it in an envelope. Remember, you want to write at least seven letters. If you want to continue giving yourself the encouragement and help that may someday prove very useful, do it.

Put your letters in your Success folder and hold them for use on a day when you feel that your success is being threatened by feelings of doubt or negative thoughts. Then go to your folder and take out a letter. It will be like a hand of friendship from your own best friend. Our wish and hope is that it will remind you of the harmony that is yours and the success, joy, and freedom that await you.

*Letter #1*

_____

_____

_____

_____

_____

_____

_____

_____

_____

_____

_____

_____

_____

_____

_____

_____

_____

_____

*Letter #2*

_____

_____

_____

_____

_____

_____

_____

_____

_____

_____

_____

_____

_____

_____

_____

_____

_____

_____

**Letter #3**

_____

_____

_____

_____

_____

_____

_____

_____

_____

_____

_____

_____

_____

_____

_____

_____

*Letter #4*

_____

_____

_____

_____

_____

_____

_____

_____

_____

_____

_____

_____

_____

_____

_____

_____

_____

_____

_____

*Letter #5*

_____

_____

_____

_____

_____

_____

_____

_____

_____

_____

_____

_____

_____

_____

_____

_____

_____

_____

_____

_____

*Letter #6*

_____

_____

_____

_____

_____

_____

_____

_____

_____

_____

_____

_____

_____

_____

_____

_____

_____

_____

*Letter #7*

_____

_____

_____

_____

_____

_____

_____

_____

_____

_____

_____

_____

_____

_____

_____

_____

_____

_____

_____

_____

_____

# CHAPTER 12

# Saying No, Saying Yes

He who refuses nothing will soon have nothing to refuse.
—Martial

## The Power of No

Saying no can mean very different things to different people. Some people say no easily, without fear or guilt. They hear a request, and if they don't want to comply, they simply say no—simply, directly, without fear of punishment or retaliation.

Some of us shrink from saying no, and will do virtually anything to avoid it. We go to comical and even tragic extremes to avoid refusing someone's request. We may resent the request or the requester, or we may make up elaborate lies or excuses—anything to avoid saying no.

---

**We have been taught to do many things—sacrifice our free time, our fun, our preferences, and our integrity—in order to avoid having to say no.**

---

Why do we behave in such foolish ways when we come face-to-face with a simple request from another person? Because to most of us, there is no such thing as a "simple" request. In the past, we have been deprived and punished by other people saying no. We have been shamed by being called "selfish" by people who wanted us to swallow our objections for their convenience. To most of us, the word *no* has become a forbidden, a "no-no." We have been taught to do many things—to sacrifice our free time, our fun, our preferences, and our integrity—in order to avoid having to say no.

## Just Beyond Arm's Reach

*Rachael:*

As a young child, I was often dependent upon my sister and brother. If I needed to reach a shelf or to open a jar, to carry something heavy or to read my favorite storybook, I was at the mercy of their much older hands and arms and minds. At any given moment, a "no" or a "not now" could cut off my access to pleasure, to entertainment, or to accomplishment. My happiness was at the whim of other people's moods. My parents were often working in the grocery store below our apartment and my brother and sister used "no" as much as a tool of vengeance as of denial.

Food was my sister's and brother's favorite venue for denying me. I was always hungry and they were always in control. I remember asking my brother to get the ice-cream sandwich my mother had left for me in the freezer. I had tried to reach it by standing on a chair, but it was just beyond arm's reach. I had even tried prying it out with a spatula but couldn't get a good angle. I was forced to ask my brother for his help. I was surprised when he didn't say "no" or "not now" but, with a pleasant look, rose and went immediately to the kitchen. "Is this what you wanted?" he asked pleasantly. I reached out my hand to the long-awaited treat.

But something was wrong. He didn't turn it over to me. Instead, he began unwrapping it. Then he took a big bite and smiled down at me. "Don't you want to share this with me?" he asked. I couldn't answer. If I said yes he would eat half my ice cream and I would hate myself for "giving in." If I said no he would eat it anyway. I can still see him standing above me and smiling as he slowly nibbled his way through it.

"I'm gonna tell," I cried. "Go ahead," he retorted. My father was out and my mother was busy covering the store alone. My report of my brother's unfairness was not well received. ". . . and he ate the whole thing himself," I finished, the tears streaming down my cheeks. Four customers were waiting to be served. "I'm busy right now," my mother said. "Besides," she added, looking down at my more-than-chunky body, "you didn't need that ice cream anyway." The first customer winked at my mother in agreement, and humiliation was added to my anger and disappointment.

Though denying me things was one of my siblings' favorite forms of entertainment, I, on the other hand, was allowed to refuse them nothing. "Rachael, go get that" or "Rachael, sit here and watch this and call me when . . ." were always ringing in the air. No matter what I was doing, my time and energy were first and foremost at their command. If any of their requests were met by my "no," they would remind me that "someday you're going to want something from me." "Just you wait" soon became a phrase that ruled my thinking.

As I grew older, my fear of saying no ruled my life. I learned to ask others for nothing. Still, I was a "giver" to the extreme. Friends and boyfriends were able to take advantage of me easily. I spoiled them with gifts and favors and asked nothing in return. Anything they asked for or seemed to need was theirs. Though I was not aware of it at the time, I was terrified to say no for fear of some unnamed reprisal. Or for fear of being abandoned. Being overweight didn't help. I told myself that I was lucky to have any friends at all. Who was I to say no?

Often, after I had forced myself to go along with what others wanted, my body would call for food to soothe the pain. I longed to have the courage to stand up for myself, but I could not say no to them and I could not say no to myself. I would call myself names and blame myself for not standing up to them. I saw myself as a coward and ate to soothe that pain as well. The heavier I became, the less likely I was to say no to anyone. Long, very long after I no longer needed them, my sister's and my brother's lessons still ruled my life.

Many years and many moments of truth later, I have faced my fears and have found the courage to say no. When I first met Richard, I fell totally in love with him (as I still am to this day). As I got to know him, I realized how rare and wonderful a man he was and how incredibly lucky I was to have him (as I still am to this day). Yet, as frightened as I was of losing him, the years of failure and newfound success told me that I had to find the courage to say no when I had to.

"You are number three in my life," I told Richard a few weeks after we began dating. "Number one is staying on my eating program. Keeping my weight down will always be number one on my list of priorities. Number two is my education. I have to finish my doctorate," I told him. "As much as I love you, you are number three, and if being with you interferes with number one or number two, being with you will have to go. The reason is simple. If I don't take care of my eating program and my education, I will never be able to be happy with you or with myself. So they have to come first."

That meant that there were many times I had to say no to the man I loved and valued because I knew that saying yes would mean putting aside my goals and myself and, in the end, that would make me (and him) miserable. Saying no was essential to my Circle of Success. (Richard loves to say that by helping me complete my doctorate, he has moved into the number-two spot. "But," he adds, "I'll never be number one. And that's the way it should be.")

Learning to say no is learning to put yourself first, without worrying about what people will think about you or say about you or do to you. It is an incredible freedom. Come share it with us.

## The No's from Your Past

EXPERIENCE #28: NEGATIVE MANEUVERS

Let's go back and look at the no's in your past.
Complete the following sentences:

As a child, if I was told no _____

_____

_____

If I would have argued with my parents' no's they would have __

_____

_____

_____

As an adolescent, my parents did not let me _____

_____

_____

and I felt _____

_____

Instead of directly saying no, people in my family _____

_____

_____

_____

Sometimes my parents would say no to me and yes to others. (Give details.) _____

_____

_____

_____

At those times, I felt _____

_____

_____


Now we will use these memories in the next Experience.


### EXPERIENCE #29: THE GLASS WALL

Receiving a no from someone who has the power to deny you something you want has been described as the "glass wall." You can see what you want but you have no way of getting to it.

Close your eyes. Remember some of the experiences from the last exercise, when someone's saying no stood between you and something you really wanted. It may have been related to food or to anything else you wanted.

Write down the details of what happened. What did you want? Who said no?

_____

_____

_____

_____

_____

_____

_____


Did they explain why you couldn't have what you wanted? Did they comfort you, or did they act in some other way? _____

_____

_____

_____

_____

_____

What did you feel? _____

_____

_____

_____

From that time on _____

_____

_____

_____

Soon we will ask you to write down any promises or decisions that you might have made in response to that no or to the many other no's you have experienced in your life. First, let's look at some examples of real-life stories of the impact of no's on people's lives. The decisions that came from those experiences are marked in the stories that follow.

### Michelle's Story:

When I wanted a bike, my parents explained that we didn't have a lot of money and that everything they earned went to feed and clothe us. My mother started to cry and I felt terrible. *I decided that asking for what you wanted was pretty selfish and that the bike didn't really matter so much.*

*Marge's Story:*

My family never went on vacation. My dream was to go to Disneyland, but almost any vacation would have done. Oh, we'd go to visit my mother's parents in Jersey and then we would go to the beach for two or three days. But I wanted a real vacation. I wanted to stay in a hotel and everything. Year after year my parents would promise, and each spring I'd get excited and start to ask where we were going. Each summer they would say that we would have to wait until next year because they couldn't afford it, or that it would be better to spend the time fixing up our home or something. We'd all hang around the house all summer. Sometimes I was able to get jobs being a mother's helper or a baby-sitter. I guess I felt sorry for myself for not having a "real" vacation. I'd spend my money on treats and sweets, and by the time school rolled around I was five or ten pounds heavier. My parents didn't come out and say we would never go on vacation, but my sister and I finally got the message. I guess we both learned that you can't trust it when people promise you things, so it's not worth building your hopes up. *I learned that the only good times I was going to get were the ones I gave myself, and most of those were edible.*

*Alex's Story:*

I always wanted a Red Ryder BB gun when I was a kid. I was a chubby boy and not much good at sports, but I knew that I could be good at shooting if I ever got a chance. Several of my friends had Red Ryders and my dream was to spend my Saturdays shooting tin cans and paper targets with them. I asked my parents for a Red Ryder for my birthday, but they said that I should concentrate more on my grades. They said that if I got all A's and B's they would get me one. I knew that they didn't think I could do it, but they didn't know how much I wanted the gun. I put more work into school that semester than I did for all of the rest of my school years combined. I didn't have time for anything else; I lost a lot of weight and was really looking pretty good. My work paid off. I got four A's, three B's, and one C (in gym). I tried to convince them that it still averaged out to all A's and B's, but they stuck to the letter of the deal. I hated them for the power they had to say no and the fact that there was nothing I could do about it. I didn't have it in me to try again. I turned my anger into eating and gained a good 20 pounds in the next year. On a short kid, that really showed. *I learned not to trust other people and that, if I wanted something in the future, I'd have to figure out a way to give it to myself.*

Now think about your stories and the conclusions and decisions that you made in response to your getting a no. Write them down on this page. Remember as much detail as you can and, when you are finished, write down the conclusion or decision that you made or the lesson that each experience taught you.

Experience #1: _____

_____

_____

_____

_____

The lesson I learned was _____

_____

_____

_____

Experience #2: _____

_____

_____

_____

_____

The lesson I learned was _____

_____

_____

_____

Experience #3: _____

_____

_____

_____

_____

The lesson I learned was _____

_____

_____

_____

Experience #4: _____

_____

_____

_____

The lesson I learned was _____

_____

_____

_____

If you have additional memories or if you need more room, add your own sheets of paper.

Now, just for the moment, put these responses aside and move on to the next Experience. We will bring them together as we complete the Experiences that follow.

## The No's That Remain Today

EXPERIENCE #30: CRYSTAL PRISONS

We carry the feelings that we connect to past no's with us every day, and, in very powerful ways, the lessons of our past no's continue to influence our choices today. For some of us, the glass walls of the past become crystal prisons of today, surrounding us and barring us from our Circles of Success.

Let's see how the no's of your past may still be influencing you today.

Complete the following sentences. Try to be as honest as you can; don't worry about how you think that you should act or feel. Answer as to how *you* really act or what you really feel. Don't worry about being consistent. Some of the questions may seem similar, but they may bring out different answers.

Complete these sentences:

If someone asks me to do something I don't want to do, I _____

_____

_____

If I say no to someone, _____

_____

_____


In general, people who can say no easily are _____

_____

_____


If I say no to someone I care about, *they* _____

_____

_____


If I say no to someone I care about, *I* _____

_____

_____


If someone asks me to do something I don't want to do, I _____

_____

_____


When I say no to someone in my family, I feel _____

_____

_____

When I say no to a friend, I feel _____

_____

_____

_____

When I say no to someone I don't like, I feel _____

_____

_____

It's easier for me to say no if _____

_____

_____

If someone has said no to me and then I say no to him or her, I

_____

_____

_____

I feel that it's easier for me to say no if _____

_____

_____

When I have to say no to myself, I feel _____

_____

_____

It's easier to say no to myself if _____

_____

_____

When I should say no, my mind says _____

_____

but _____

_____

Now it is time to use the no's of the past and of the present to make a far better future.

---

**The word *no* rarely means a simple denial
of a request. For most of us no means
a great deal more.**

---

The word *no* rarely means a simple denial of a request. For most of us, no means a great deal more than merely having to do without something. In childhood, a no may have made us angry because we couldn't control the situation or those around us. We may have felt powerless and frustrated, or, even worse, controlled by other people. We may have learned to associate no with a feeling of being unloved or unimportant; no may have been used to punish us or to tell us that we were bad.

It is no wonder that so many of us avoid it as adults. We delay, fib, finagle, compromise, and often do what we clearly don't want to do, in order to avoid saying (or hearing) yet another no.

**We delay, fib, finagle, compromise, and often do
what we clearly don't want to do, in order to
avoid saying (or hearing) yet another no.**

## EXPERIENCE #31: THE CLOUDED REFLECTION

Now it's time to look over your responses to the last two Experiences in order to see how the no's of your past are still influencing your feelings today. Look at the responses in the Experience before the last, "The Glass Wall." Read over your own responses to "The Lesson I Learned Was," the lines that you underlined. Read your responses aloud so that you will really hear them. Don't judge them; they reflect your experiences, and you have a right to feel the way you do.

After you have finished reading the responses aloud, look at the section that you just completed, "Crystal Prisons." Read these sentences aloud, too. Look for the connections that are almost sure to connect between your no's Past and your no's Present. For example, when confronted with no's in the past, did you carry with you the idea that to be told no meant that you were bad, or selfish, or demanding? Did you feel ashamed or self-centered or a bother to other people? If so, you probably now assume that others will feel the same way if you say no to them. No wonder you find it hard to say no.

As a child you may have been given the message that when someone makes a request it is, in reality, a demand, not something that you can really refuse. You may have come to accept the idea that, although it may look like you have choice, the truth is, you don't.

If you were made to feel ashamed of wanting things for yourself, you may have concluded that to want things is selfish. When people make requests of you now, you probably don't know how to refuse them, since that would involve putting your wishes first. Many people find that their emotional responses to requests are out of proportion to the matter at hand; they feel put-upon and confused at the same time, afraid to simply say no.

If, in the past, you were not told directly that you couldn't have something or if promises were not always kept, you may have come to the conclusion that you can't rely on people or trust them to keep their word. When people ask you for something now, you may overcompensate by giving them what they want, however unreasonable or inconvenient, for fear of breaking the trust as others did to you.

---

**While the present reflects the past, it is an image clouded by a child's view and by the feelings of pain and powerlessness that often go along with being young.**

---

While the present reflects the past, it is an image clouded by a child's view and by the feelings of pain and powerlessness that often go along with being young.

Read aloud your responses to No's Past and Present and see and feel the connections between what you experienced in the past and what you still believe and feel now. Write them down below.

_____

_____

_____

_____

_____

_____

_____

_____

_____

_____

_____

_____

_____

_____

_____

_____

_____

_____

## EXPERIENCE #32: HOW DO YOU RESPOND TO A NO?

Check off all of the words that you associate with feelings about being told no:

| | | |
|---|---|---|
| ___ anger | ___ punishment | ___ revenge |
| ___ withholding | ___ powerlessness | ___ rage |
| ___ control | ___ deprivation | ___ frustration |
| ___ lack of interest | ___ unfairness | ___ rejection |
| ___ guilt | ___ distress | ___ nastiness |
| ___ hate | ___ pain | ___ loneliness |
| ___ defiance | ___ hopelessness | ___ tyranny |
| ___ fury | ___ sadness | ___ depression |
| ___ rebellion | ___ opposition | ___ disapproval |
| ___ sadism | ___ badness | ___ shame |
| ___ humiliation | ___ selfishness | ___ guilt |

SCORING YOUR RESPONSE TO NO'S:

**0–7:** Your probably have had your share of no's in your past, but you have been able to find your way around them. When you come face-to-face with a no, you look for other ways to get what you want anyway. You don't spend a great deal of time trying to change the situation; you look for other means to get what you need.

**8–17:** The no's of your past still have an impact on you today. You respond to being denied things strongly, though you are usually able, in time, to move on to getting what you want by some other means. The unfairness of situations and people bothers you, and you may spend more time than you think wise trying to make them see things "your way."

**18–30:** You hate to get a no, and your emotional response to them can keep you from making the best choices. You may lose your temper, or, at times, feel totally unmotivated. You do well when you are encouraged but have a great deal of difficulty when you encounter resistance. At times you may tell yourself that it's no use or there's no use in trying. The no's that you have experienced in the past are difficult to overcome.

### Chuck's Story:

When she announced the arrival of Chuck S. at our office, our secretary had a glint in her eye. "Your next appointment is here," she informed us and, without compromising her professional manner, managed to communicate that she found him very attractive.

Chuck was struggling with 20 extra pounds, a strong addiction to carbohydrates that overpowered him in the evenings, and the inability to say no to his ex-wife, Sharon. He was, nevertheless, engaging and good-looking.

When his wife left him for another man, Chuck moved to a one-room apartment nearby, but continued to take care of what soon became "her" home and car. After she and the children left the house, he would go in and do the necessary home repair and maintenance that his ex-wife requested. When she said that she had trouble picking up the children after school, Chuck arranged his schedule so that he could pick them up, help them with their homework, and feed them a hot meal before he went back to work. He regularly stayed at his job long into the evening to put in the hours that he had missed in order to accede to his wife's requests.

Chuck himself would often pick up food on the run, grabbing whatever was easy and handy. Dieting became impossible because it required that he put himself first. His weight was going up and his cravings for snack foods and candy were increasing by the day.

"I don't feel like I have time to *think,* much less to follow a diet. I'm always on the run, and it seems like the more I do, the more remains undone. No matter what I do, it's not good enough, and Sharon is always asking for more. I know she's taking advantage of me, but I can't seem to say no."

In order to help Chuck stay on an eating program that would reduce his cravings and weight, we first had to help him discover what was standing between him and his denying his ex-wife whatever she wanted.

We encouraged him to answer the open-ended statements that you have been working with in this chapter. This is what he remembered about a very important "no" in his life:

"I was seventeen, just starting my last year in high school. I wanted to borrow money to buy insurance for a car. I said that I would work for the money for the car and asked my parents if they would lend me the money for the insurance. I explained that I could use the car to deliver pizza and maybe make enough money to pay them back and have spending money of my own.

"After I told them what I wanted and why I wanted it, my parents just kind of looked at each other and told me they would think about it. I had already asked my mother for the money, but she had said no. She told me that she didn't want me to work on school nights and was afraid that I would get into a car accident. My father wanted me to get a job and resented giving me an allowance at my age. I knew that they disagreed, but I asked for the money anyway.

"They argued for almost a week. I tried to tell them that I would figure out some other way to get a job, but the arguments continued. I can still remember the screaming.

"My mother wanted to say no and my father wouldn't let her. My father finally won out and said that he would lend me the money whenever I wanted, but I never asked him for the loan again. I was terrified that the fighting would start all over. I figured that nothing that I wanted was worth the fighting and the screaming. I felt guilty and selfish for bringing it up when I knew they disagreed in the first place, and I told myself that I should have taken my mother's no for an answer."

Chuck's fear of saying no to his ex-wife was tied up with his experiences as a child. His ex-wife used his fear of saying no to his children to get whatever she wanted out of him. Whenever she sensed that he was about to refuse her anything, she would make the request on behalf of the kids. When she did, Chuck was a goner. His work, his money, his diet and health and his life, were all put on hold in order to avoid saying no.

When he came to see us, Chuck had started dating a woman who seemed like a wonderful choice, but as her demands on his time became greater, Chuck was caught between saying no to her or to his ex-wife. His eating patterns and his weight reflected Chuck's conflict. He had put on 10 pounds in the last month, he told us, about twice what he had put on in the two months before. His eating was out of control, his weight was out of control, and his life was out of control—all because he didn't know how to say no.

Six months and a great deal of good hard work later, Chuck had shed 22 pounds and his ex-wife's control as well. After remembering his parents' fight, Chuck had taken a good hard look at himself. He learned to say no with a clear and resounding finality. He backed it up with a lawyer's advice and put his energy into developing an independent relationship with his children.

He had shared his memory of his parents' fighting with Sandy, his soon-to-be fiancée. She listened with loving care, and as she came to understand that Chuck's difficulties did not reflect a lessening of his affection for her, she was able to help him deal with his doubts and fears. "She is the best thing that ever happened to me," he said to us. "And I almost lost her because of the fears of a guilty seventeen-year-old."

It's been over two years now. Chuck and Sandy are married. They spend weekends and vacation time with Chuck's children, and

Sandy is expecting a child. Chuck's weight and eating are easily managed and his life is "better than I ever thought it could be."

"Saying no used to be the hardest thing in the world for me. It's still not easy, but I can do it when I have to. For the first time in my life, I feel like my own person," he says.

## Saying No and Saying Yes in the Future

EXPERIENCE #33: THE POWER TO CHOOSE TO SAY NO

The past leads to the present and the present to the future. Looking at what we have experienced and felt can lead us to understand what we now believe and what we feel. But the wonderful part of being alive and growing is that we are uniquely able to change our future.

Take all of the pages that have made up your responses to the Experiences in this chapter and destroy them. They are related to old pain that has kept you prisoner long enough. Burn them or tear them up. Destroy them totally. The insights that you have gained go far beyond words. You carry them in the deepest parts of you and will need no reminder in the future. Let go and move on.

---

*No* is a powerful word, but we can learn to use
it in order to grow strong and healthy. It is
only by being able to choose to say no to others
when we want that we find the time and energy
and right to say yes to ourselves.

---

It is time to learn to say no without blame or guilt, sensitively and with love. We can separate the pain that we have so long coupled with hearing or saying no, and we can come to say no as a statement of strength and resolve.

Read each of the following sentences aloud. Circle those that you want to use in the future in order to be able to say no to others. Keep them handy in your Success folder and read them over whenever you like. They are friends that will help you change the patterns that have held you captive for so long. As you think of other sentences of your own, write them in the spaces that follow.

Here are *new* ways of saying no that do not carry the blame and pain of the past. You may want to use them when you really want to say no but don't have the words:

> "I really would rather not. I need some time to myself."

> "That's not something that I feel comfortable doing. Maybe we can think of something different."

> "I've been spending a lot of time away from the house (or family). I really need time to catch up."

> "I really can't make the time right now. I'm overloaded. I'm sorry."

> "I can see that you're upset, but I really need to say no right now."

> "I'm sorry, but I'd rather not."

Write down any sentences of your own that came to mind when you read these sentences. Keep your sentences simple statements of preference. Don't overexplain or defend yourself. Saying no may be difficult, but all of us must finally learn that we may choose, at times, to say no.

_____

_____

_____

_____

_____

_____

## EXPERIENCE #34: THE POWER TO CHOOSE TO SAY YES

If learning to say no is difficult, one would expect that saying yes should be easy. Not so. Saying yes to ourselves (not others) often must be learned. The same guilt that accompanies a no to others may go along with giving permission to ourselves.

Saying no to others can sometimes translate as a yes to ourselves. "No, I can't help out right now" means "Yes, I will have time to do my own work." "No, I don't agree" means "Yes, I do have my own opinion."

It seems easy, but yes's, when directed to ourselves, often elude the best of us. We often do not take the time and trouble to make ourselves comfortable or to give ourselves pleasure or even to keep ourselves healthy.

In the spaces which follow, list the things that you would like to say yes to for yourself. It may be taking the time to enjoy a nap, preparing a special food that you love, a long overdue visit to the doctor, a vacation that you could probably afford but cannot get yourself to commit to, or even the time to go to the bathroom when the urge makes itself known.

Post this sheet in a place where you can see it and be reminded of the yeses that need to be said to yourself. Day after day, week after week, check off each yes that means that you are learning to take care of yourself. As additional wants make themselves known, write them down and give them to yourself. Sometimes it's good to just say yes.

Yes (✓) _____

Yes (✓) _____

Yes (✓) _____

Yes (✓) _____

Yes (✓) _____

Yes (✓) _____

Yes (✔) _____

Yes (✔) _____

Yes (✔) _____

Yes (✔) _____

Yes (✔) _____

Yes (✔) _____

Yes (✔) _____

Yes (✔) _____

Yes (✔) _____

Yes (✔) _____

Yes (✔) _____

Yes (✔) _____

Yes (✔) _____

Yes (✔) _____

Yes (✔) _____

Yes (✔) _____

Yes (✔) _____

Yes (✔) _____

Yes (✔) _____

Yes (✔) _____

Yes (✔) _____

# CHAPTER 13

# Your Own Private Dream

We are such stuff as dreams are made on.

—Shakespeare

## The Fragile Flower

A dream is a very private thing. It grows far from the harsh light of close examination and blooms for only very short periods of time. It must be nurtured with unstinting hope and childlike trust. Above all, it must be protected against ridicule or it will quickly wither and die.

Children are taught, all too soon, to hide their dreams far from the view of others. They learn to "act mature," to "be reasonable" and "practical." Years go by and hidden dreams may be forever lost.

## A Dream Delayed, a Dream Come True

*Richard:*

Even as a teenager, I had a dream of sharing my life with the "ideal" woman. She didn't have to be beautiful in the classical sense, but in my dreams, she was radiant. Her figure was unimportant to me—that's never been an issue in my life—though I pictured her as healthy and strong and confident.

I envisioned my body as powerful, muscular, and proud. I saw

**229**

myself as agile and free and perfectly slender as we sailed effortlessly, like two graceful ice-skaters, across the rink. I longed for the
two of us to fly free with our minds and our bodies. She would
bring out the best in me; I would do the same for her. We would
laugh and talk and make love, without self-consciousness or concern. We would work together and do great things for all the world
to see. I imagined us moving through life, sharing our thoughts, our
feelings, and our energies. In perfect sync, we would flow together.

---

**My real life was far from that dream. . . .
I lived a life of quiet desperation.**

---

My real life was far from that dream. My extra thirty pounds were
a deep and disturbing issue to me though I never discussed it. I felt
that my inability to control my eating and weight reflected some
deeper lack within me. I lived in fear of the weight gain and the
health problems that were sure to come as I grew older. My personal life felt like a series of chores and duties. The only joy that I
knew was in the laughter of my children. My dream had been silenced by my dismal reality. As I look back at it now, I can see that
I lived a life of quiet desperation.

---

**My dream, though silenced for so long, never died.
When my marriage dissolved after sixteen years,
my fantasy of a joyful and creative relationship
re-emerged, innocent, golden, and shining.**

---

When I saw couples who seemed truly to enjoy each other, I
would tell myself that they were "showing off," or to comfort myself, I would knowingly smile and say that it would all change after
a few years of marriage. But my dream, though silenced for so long,
never died, and when my marriage dissolved after sixteen years, my
fantasy of a joyful and creative relationship re-emerged, innocent,
golden, and shining.

I told friends that I did not see my divorce as a loss but rather
as a chance to reach for the happiness that had eluded me. They
patted me gently on the back and tried to tell me that I was denying
my pain. Colleagues sought to console me on the breakup of my

marriage. I shared my excitement at this unforseen opportunity to capture the joy and freedom that I had all but stopped hoping for. They gave me their home phone numbers in case I needed help when I got "in touch" with my feelings.

As the dog days of divorce courts and lawyers dragged on, my weight plummeted. I found myself free to eat in the way that *I* knew resulted in fewer cravings and easy weight loss for *me*. I was able to follow the eating plan that I had long suspected would work for me. The 30 pounds dropped away easily and effortlessly.

I looked great, I felt great, and what is more, for the first time in many, many years, my dream was alive.

Within five weeks, my dream had come true. Slim and secure in my own knowledge of my body and my control of my eating, I met Rachael. She was all that I dreamed of and more. Although she carried with her a lifetime of love never appreciated and pain never discarded, she, too, carried the Dream. I brought the rules of a failed relationship and financial burdens that seemed overwhelming. The flow of love and creativity we share today is genuine and real and the result of many hours of sharing and crying and learning together, but most of all, it is the result of *two* people who both sought the joy and freedom that others saw as foolish.

Seven years later, we continue to live the dream. It didn't come as soon as I thought it would, or as easily. In the beginning we would sit long into the night and explore the bruises and scars we still carried from the past so that we could leave them behind and enjoy our lives together. Fewer hurts emerge these days, but when they do, they are tended with patient, loving care.

We are together twenty-four hours a day, rarely more than five feet apart. We teach in the medical school together, we write together, we lecture and conduct our research at the Center, side by side. We never get tired of each other. Our eating patterns, sleeping patterns, love of music and life are identical. Our purpose in life is the same. Our respect and appreciation of each other is constant. We work hard and play hard, but we never fail to make time for each other. We share every aspect of our lives, but of all of these, the most important thing we share is the Dream.

## Dreams Denied

Sometimes dreams fight back. They want to be known and to be heard. When your dreams are ignored they may pinch you to remind you of their existence. Pinches can come as sweet longings: with a spring day, a summer evening, or the smell of cologne, an ache wells up inside.

Don't be fooled when you see someone acting in a surprisingly cold and determined manner, exhibiting a no-nonsense attitude, a brusque, businesslike approach to life. All of these can be the outward expression of a sweet, soft dream being jammed back down below the surface. Some reminders of the dream hurt, as we find ourselves feeling weepy or blue for "no reason." We have no zest, no interest in almost anything. If we are lucky enough to have an understanding friend, or if we take the time to listen to ourselves, we may discover that our sadness comes from a dream crying to be heard.

When time passes and dreams remain unfulfilled, they can become a catchall for any new pain or disappointment that comes along. Perhaps you dream of having an attractive, slender, healthy body, but you never get a chance to make your dream a reality. With each new disappointment, your desire may escalate into a craving to have the the sexiest body imaginable. No more will a pleasant shape do; your compensatory fantasy may now include seducing movie stars and marrying multimillionaires. Gone are the simple days of wishing for an end to a protruding tummy or cellulite-ridden thighs; now nothing less than fame, fortune, and adventure will meet your needs.

Soon, past disappointments and everyday problems join forces and seek relief in an all-encompassing dream of escape. "Someday I'm just going to walk out that door and never come back. I'm going to put some money aside, and one day, I'm going to just disappear very quietly, on my own." When we hear this dream, we hear far more than a desire to get away. We hear the pain of many other dreams that have never been realized. We remember the many times when the needs of others were put first. We hear echoes of the disappointments, unkept promises, lack of interest, and enforced loneliness that led to the necessity of a dream of escape.

Dreams of escape and compensatory dreams are dreams denied.

Dreams are the expression of emotional longings, and like many emotions, whether anger or fear or resentment, they can be contained for a while, but will not be forgotten. Sooner or later they will make themselves known.

When we make our daily dreams come true, compensatory and escape dreams usually fade. When escape dreams do remain, however, they may be saying that it is, indeed, time to move on to a more fulfilling and happy future.

At the Carbohydrate Addict's Center, we recommend that our participants complete the Experiences that follow in this chapter. Almost everyone comes in with dreams of one kind or another. Some people never share their dreams; some demand on-the-spot dream fulfillment. Most people know intuitively that dreams are important to listen to and understand. Dreams guide us. They are the letter paper of our hearts.

It's time to remember your dreams and to breathe life into them once again. First let's look at the dreams of yesterday and today, sorting the reachable dreams from the unreachable. Then we'll work toward making your own best dreams a waking, breathing reality.

## Your Dreams Past

### EXPERIENCE #35: YOUNG DREAMS

Complete the sentences that follow. If a sentence does not seem to apply to you, leave it blank and move on to the next.

1.  When I was a child, I dreamed that I would _____

    _____

    _____

    By the age of nine or ten or eleven, I dreamed that I would

    _____

    _____

As a teenager, I dreamed that I would _____

_____

_____

_____

2. One wish that I told to no one (or almost no one) was _____

_____

_____

3. As a youngster, the closest I ever came to having a wish come

    true was _____

    _____

    _____

    and I felt _____

4. As a child, if I had three wishes I would have wished for:

    Wish #1 _____

    Wish #2 _____

    Wish #3 _____

5. If I could reach back in time, and grant the child that I was one

    wish, it would be: _____

_____

_____

6. If someone would have made that one dream come true for me

   as a child, _____

   _____

   _____

   _____

7. When I was younger, I thought dreams _____

   _____

Don't do anything with these answers for the moment. For now, move on to the next Experience.

## Your Dreams Today

**EXPERIENCE #36: NEW DREAMS**

1. To this day I still dream of _____

   _____

   _____

2. One wish that I have told to no one (or almost no one) is ___

   _____

   _____

3.  As an adult, the closest I ever came to having a wish come true

    was _____

    _____

    and I felt _____

4.  If I had three wishes today I would wish for:

    Wish #1 _____

    Wish #2 _____

    Wish #3 _____

5.  If, right now, I could grant myself one wish, it would be ____

    _____

    _____

6.  If I could make this dream come true, _____

    _____

    _____

7.  As an adult, I think dreams _____

    _____

    _____

Let's see how your dreams have stood the test of time. Look at each sentence you completed in "Your Dreams Past" and compare it to the corresponding sentence in "Your Dreams Today."

As you compare your Young Dreams (Past) with your New Dreams (Present), think about these questions:

Have your dreams remained the same? Don't be fooled by this one. Dreams may look different but may be expressing the same desire. If, as a child, you wanted to become a fireman or a nurse and today you dream of discovering a cure for cancer, you may be expressing the same dream. Look to the purpose of the dream. In this case, it's a desire to help other people. On the other hand, you might have wanted to be a nurse as a child so that you could help people, and want to be a nurse today because it provides good pay, flexible hours, and security. Although the dreams appear to be the same, they are expressing two different purposes and are two different dreams.

Look at the secrecy that you associate with your dreams. Did you keep them to yourself as a child? Do you still protect them? Why? How do you think secrecy affects the probability that you can achieve your dreams? Would you share your dreams in order to ask for help? As a child, what did you think would happen if other people knew about your dreams? Has your attitude changed? Is (was) there reason to believe that this is (was) true?

How does it feel to have a dream come true? Has that feeling changed over time? If it has changed, why do you think that feeling changed?

Have your "three wishes" changed? Remember, look beyond the surface to the purpose of the wish. If your wishes have changed, how have they changed? What changed them? What remained the same?

Which dreams were never fulfilled in childhood? Which remain today? Are they the same?

Has your view of dreams, and of dreaming, changed? Would your answer be different if more of your dreams had come true? How does that make you feel? If it does not make you feel good, what could you do now to get what you want?

EXPERIENCE #37: ARE YOU A DOUBTING DREAMER?

Many of us dream in halfway measures. "It can't hurt," we tell ourselves, whereas another part of us says, "Yeah, but it can't help either."

By the time we get to adulthood, most of us have pretty much given up on dreaming. Oh, we hold on to a fantasy or two, a "wouldn't it be lovely if . . ." kind of thought, but we don't put too much stock in it. Chances are, the most we do to try and make our dreams come true is to buy a lottery ticket and cross our fingers.

We want to believe. It would be great if believing in dreams made them come true. But the truth is that we don't see any proof that dreaming works. So we largely give up on dreaming, except for a secret hope way down deep inside, and adjust our thinking to go along with our more "realistic" view. But if bread is the staff of life for our bodies, dreaming is the staff of life for our souls. It nurtures us, sustains us, and gives us the strength to go on.

At times our minds, in conflict with our feelings, make judgments about our dreaming and leave us feeling embarrassed, even ashamed, of wanting our dreams to come true. One part of us carries the vision of life as it could be; another part of us crushes that hope with an unfeeling coldness. It may even taunt us and make us feel ashamed of the desires we hold most dear.

The result is a Doubting Dreamer—one who carries the hope and beauty within but whose mind disallows the fantasy of the fulfillment.

Let's see if you are a Doubting Dreamer. Check off *any and all* of the following that reflect your beliefs.

| **COLUMN A** | **COLUMN B** |
|---|---|
| *Dreams:* | *Dreams:* |

|  |  |
|---|---|
| ___ are important | ___ are silly |
| ___ can be more enjoyable than reality | ___ only make us unhappy |
| ___ help us to reach for more | ___ are a waste of time |
| ___ are important for everyone | ___ are only for children |
| ___ must be shared | ___ are best kept to yourself |
| ___ keep you from doing what needs to get done | ___ keep you focused on your goals |

Now compare your answers in Column A with those in Column B. Each line reflects opposite views about dreams. Some of us hold beliefs on both sides at the same time; this is the sign of the Doubting Dreamer.

If you had checks on the same line in both columns, or if you had an approximately equal number of checks in Column A and Column B, you probably feel conflicted about letting yourself dream. The greater number of same-line checks, the greater your conflict. Doubts about allowing yourself to dream, and making those dreams come true, can cause conflict to tear apart your Circle of Success. When you are in doubt, your feelings fight each other and pull away from the center. No matter how the other parts of you try to keep the Circle together, they cannot. (All checks in Column B confirm that you do not feel that dreaming is a positive experience but you do not appear to be in conflict).

If you are a Doubting Dreamer, take a good look at the reasons for your conflicted feelings. Doubting Dreamers are usually disappointed dreamers in disguise. When dreams don't come true, it's easy to stop believing. But it is then that you *must* keep believing. There are so many times when we are tempted to give up but when, because we persevere, our dreams come true. Life has a myriad of surprises; we never know what will happen next. We cannot afford to let our dreams die, for if they do, the opportunity to make them come true slips through our fingers.

*Rachael:*

Eleven years ago I weighed 300 pounds. I had only my high school diploma and worked at two jobs that, together, barely kept a roof over my head. I lived in a single-room occupancy hotel, infested with mice and roaches, and I had a total of twenty dollars in the bank. I was in a relationship that was turning abusive, but I felt so badly about myself that I could not bring myself to leave. I was going blind in one eye from a brain tumor, but I did not have the money for the operation. Everywhere I turned I faced a wall twelve feet high. My parents and brother were dead, and I had no place to turn. In an effort to get the money, I asked my boss for an advance for the doctor's fee. He fired me.

Eleven years later, I wear size six. I keep my weight off struggle-free. I have my bachelors degree, two masters, and a doctorate. I am a professor in one of the finest medical schools and one of the best graduate schools in the country. I have a city apartment and a country home. I am in fine health, active and energetic. I am the co-author of a *New York Times* bestseller along with two other books that have helped over a quarter million people to conquer the addiction we share. I am codirector of a center that helps people who have all but given up hope. Best of all, I share it with a man who loves, values, and respects me, who knows me and appreciates me, and who also knows the value of dreaming. I live a life that, yes, I *did* dream of.

---

**I kept my dreams alive and they did the
same for me.**

---

It was the dreaming and the unwillingness to give up the dream that got me where I am today. Sure, there were times that I almost let go, but the voice inside me would not be shamed or ridiculed or argued into silence. I kept my dreams alive and they did the same for me.

Often, our dreams do not come true because we sit back and wait for a miracle to happen. A Middle Eastern proverb says, "Trust in your dreams, but tie your camel anyway." If you stop believing that your dreams will come true, you stop doing your part. When you stop doing your part, the chances decrease that your dream will indeed come true. The failure of your dream to come true becomes what is called a "self-fulfilling prophecy" because it is you yourself who makes the belief (or in this case, the lack of belief) come true. It is easy to hold a dream for a moment, but what sets the winners apart from all the rest is their tenacity—their unwillingness to let go of their dreams and their willingness to do whatever must be done to make those dreams come true. It is that kind of conviction, that committment, that will make your dream come true. Hold on and don't let go. It's your dream. It's your life.

Sometimes dreams do not come true because we take no for an answer too quickly. "I tried my best," we tell ourselves. "What could I do?" we ask. Then we shrug our shoulders and walk away. We may have appeased the judge within us, but there is more to life than being judged "not guilty." Sometimes the *only* way to get what we want is to try and try and try again. If we cannot get it from one person, we have to find out who else can help us. If this turns out to be a wrong turn, we have to back up and try a different direction. Success does not come from traveling in straight lines. The path is full of twists and turns, but the only way to make your dream come true is to keep trying . . . and learning . . . and trying again.

The most successful people we have met had three things in common:

1. A deep and powerful belief that dreams do come true,
2. The willingness to put in whatever work was necessary to make it happen.
3. The unwillingness to take no for an answer.

These attributes make an unbeatable threesome that result in a tight and harmonious Circle of Success, and each is a necessary part of the whole.

There is a misconception that successful people are practical and purposeful and that being powerful and purposeful means having no time for dreams. This misconception misses the point that the drive behind successful people's actions is the dreams themselves. Without the dream there is no purpose. Successful people know it and they live it. You deserve no less.

## Your Future Dreams

EXPERIENCE #38: DREAMS OF TOMORROW

Our dreams give us joy when we are sad, comfort in our pain, and hope when we feel hopeless. They nourish our spirit, calm our bodies, and fill our minds with the wonders of what can be. They challenge us and make us keenly aware of our own shortcomings. They are the reason to keep trying when our bodies and our minds want to give up. Your dreams guide you, chide you, and never let you rest easy. They bring all parts of you together and, most of all, they give life meaning.

This Experience is the final one in this book, and the most challenging. It will call for you to summon up your courage and to get in touch with the things that *you* want. Wanting is not easy; it is the first thing that we know as a baby and the first thing we are taught to disregard as a young child. In our "civilized society," what *you* want is the last thing that you are expected to seek. The taboo against wanting reaches deep inside of us and makes us feel ashamed of having desires and hopes and goals and needs. But attaining our dreams, fulfilling our wants, are what make us happy . . . and whole.

To be truly successful, to reach for all that life has to offer, it is essential that you welcome your dreams and pay attention to those things that *you* want for *you*.

Destroy the Experiences that you have completed in this chapter; they are old dreams, dreams of conflict, dreams of another era. You have fresh dreams, new dreams, dreams of tomorrow.

Fill in the each of the following pages with as much detail as you can give. The more detail, the clearer the dream. And the clearer the dream, the closer the reality.

Complete your Dream Sheets and place them in your Success folder. Come back to visit them often. Like old friends, they will bring you harmony and joy and be glad to hear of all that you have done.

## Your Dream Sheets

Take this sheet and a pen and stand in front of a mirror. Look into the mirror.

Close your eyes. Feel yourself grow tired and cold. When you open your eyes you will see a seventy-five-year-old face looking back. It is you. Your life is coming to a close. The choices have all been made. Answer the questions that the face in the mirror now asks:

What have you done with your life? _____

_____

_____

_____

Was it a good life? _____

What were you most proud of? _____

_____

_____

What would you have done differently? _____

_____

_____

Do you consider yourself successful? _____

_____

How do you know? _____

_____

_____

Which dreams did you fulfill? _____

_____

_____

Which dreams will never come to be? _____

_____

_____

Why? _____

_____

_____

If you had more time, what would you change about your life?

_____

_____

Now, close your eyes and let warmth and vitality flow through you. Open your eyes and face yourself as you are now.

Today, you still have choice. Today, you still have time. Today, you still have a chance to make your dreams come true. It may not be easy. It may not be fast. As they say, there are no guarantees in life. But right now, you have the chance. That's more than you'll have . . . then.

Go ahead. Make it happen. Make it happen now. It is your dream. It waits for you. Only you will make it come true.

# PART V

---

# COMPLETING THE CIRCLE

# CHAPTER 14

# You Are Never Alone

## Our Readers' Own Stories

Dear Drs. Heller:

I am a very grateful reader and dieter. I am 45 years old, female, married with two grown children, a teacher, and have had a weight problem since I can remember. When I was very young, I never was terribly overweight, but my mother had to buy my clothes in the "chubby" section. Through high school, I was usually a size 18. When I was a senior in high school, I went on my first diet. I weighed 180 pounds and was a size 18. My mother took me to a doctor who prescribed Escatrol, one of the "speed"-type diet pills. I lost 20 pounds and was a motor mouth. After several weeks, as you may expect, the pills started losing their effect in the middle of the day. Fortunately, I never went back to the doctor, so I never became "hooked." Needless to say, I gained the weight back, plus more. To shorten the story, I will say that for the next 27 years I dieted, gained, dieted, gained, etc., and had two children.

In November 1991, I had been totally out of control for several months (having lost 48 pounds in 1990), and was feeling frustrated and ineffective—again. By now, my weight was well over 300. One day, in November, I happened to be free during the day, and I turned on the "Jenny Jones" show. I *never* watch daytime TV; I had never watched "Jenny Jones." But this time I did, and there you two were, talking about yet another diet. But this one sounded different.

It was meaningful that Rachael had lost 150 pounds and kept it off. It was meaningful that you were both well-educated people, in fields that lent credibility to what you were saying. I bought your book [The Carbohydrate Addict's Diet]. I took the test and found out that I was severely addicted. I actually felt relieved. It meant perhaps it wasn't my fault, that I am not a weakling who has no willpower.

I started on the diet the next day. Wow! What a difference! I went all the way through Christmas season on the diet, never "cheating." I don't have to cheat, I have my Reward meal every day. Anyway, I have no idea how much I have lost. I bought a professional scale that has a 350-pound capacity, and I weighed more than that! I was shocked and devastated! Now, however, I can weigh myself on the scale, so I know that I've lost.

The main thing I want to say, is thank you for discovering and developing the diet. I feel like Martin Luther King, Jr., since I want to say "Free at last! Free at last! Thank God Almighty, I'm free at last!" I now say with confidence, *"When I get to normal weight . . ."* I know it will happen. I know I can follow this diet for the rest of my life. Thank you, thank you, thank you!

> Sincerely,
> Catherine Greer
> Riverside, CA

Dear Drs. Heller:

Just a short note to tell you of my success with your fabulous diet. I am 71 years old, and have numerous diet failures previously. I have now lost 25 pounds, feeling great, and hope to lose another 6 pounds. I foresee no problem in doing that. . . .

> Adam Quandt
> Palmdale, CA

Dear Drs. Heller:

I am writing to tell you how much I appreciate your *Carbohydrate Addict's Diet*. I purchased the book after a friend watched the special you had on television. . . .

After 4 days on the carbohydrate addict's program, I could feel the cravings leave me. It was amazing. I could even tell you exactly what I had eaten for the last week. Prior to this program, I couldn't tell you exactly what I had eaten during the last few hours. I started the program on June 9, 1991, and I have lost 27 pounds. I feel wonderful and am looking forward to reaching my goal of 60 pounds. I am losing very slowly, but for the first time in my life I have no fear of gaining it back. . . .

I just want to let you know that this program is working for me. Also, my friend, Kathy Nelson, is also still on the program and has lost 20 pounds. . . .

Kathy Withrow
Lebanon, OR

Dear Richard and Rachael Heller:

I so very much wanted to reach you by phone yesterday afternoon when you were in Minneapolis and on WCCO radio. A dear friend of mine heard you originally back in April when you first appeared on Ruth Koslack's radio show talking about your book. Since April 23, 1991, I have been on your diet and to date have lost 64 pounds! I wanted to be able to tell you thank you for this miracle in my life. But the lines were busy and I could not get through to you.

For the first time in my life I feel I am not on a diet. I plan to eat in this manner for the rest of my life—happily, indeed. It is as though a bad switch has been thrown, and I am now running on "normal." I am so impressed by your wanting to share this wonderful news with so many people—all for the price of your book—rather than, as others have often done, by being available only to those who could afford to pay a substantial amount of money and come to some clinic. You have changed my life and I am grateful. I am not hungry, as you know, and have long since given up my guilt about eating what "normal" people do, and greatly enjoy my bread and dessert and feel no guilt at all. . . . This is now my way of life, and I have not gone off the plan once. Of course, it is now obvious that something has happened to me, and when people question me, I simply tell them I had a chemical imbalance in my body that has now been corrected. I want to shout out to the world, "I am now normal." . . .

Again, thank you, thank you, a million times, for making this wonderful plan available to anyone and everyone. If I were to see you in person, I would feel the need to give you both a big hug. Consider yourselves hugged!

> Lois M. Collings
> Edina, MN

Dear Drs. Heller:

Thank you! I purchased your book about six weeks ago and have been following the Carbohydrate Addict's Diet since. I'm truly amazed at the results so far. Most important, I feel like I have hope for the first time in years. Everything in your book is true to me. I felt like I was reading my life story. I *know* that in just a few short months I will be at a good weight and I *know* it will stay that way for the rest of my life. I'm 32 years old with a wonderful husband and four children. After having the children you can accurately guess what happened to my weight, the struggle to take it off and the ensuing frustrations of the constant failure. I had given up. I have control now. What a wonderful feeling. Thank you again! . . .

I'm not doing this plan alone. My sister and a good friend are sharing this wonderful experience as well. . . . We are so enthusiastic about this program we feel like shouting from the rooftops. . . .

> Colleen O'Shea-Moran
> Parma Heights, OH

Dear Drs. Heller:

You don't know me but I had to write you to tell you how much your book *The Carbohydrate Addict's Diet* has changed my life.

Last fall I was watching a new program called "Cover-to-Cover" when I saw you discussing your book. I took the partial test that was given on the program and I answered yes to every question. I didn't do anything then. I guess I was afraid this would be another diet program aimed to take my money and not help me. . . .

I'm 33 years old and I weighed over 270 (my scale only goes to 270) so I really don't know how much more. I have been overweight all my life. At the age of 13 I weighed 202 pounds. My mother took me to the doctor. He promptly gave me a diet and diet pills with a long lecture on how I should have more willpower. I lost 40 pounds in 7 months then he took me off the pills. In three short months I gained back 30 pounds. This has been my story ever since. I would lose weight and gain back even more. Twenty years and two children later, here I am at 270+ pounds. It took me until 1992 before I could bring myself to go to the bookstore to look at your book. I opened it to the test and took it right in the store. I was borderline between a moderate and a severe addiction.

I started the diet January 6, 1992. My life has not been the same since. I am no longer depressed. I don't crave food anymore. My energy level has come up. I can sleep better. Even better yet, that willpower the doctor lectured me on is mine. I can say no when I'm tempted. Finally I found the answer to my question, Why can't I stop eating?

As of this date I have lost 24 pounds, and I've found myself free of all pain and the terrible cravings. I feel like a new person. Thank you! In my doctor's words at my checkup, "I haven't seen you more peaceful in 12 years."

Christine Ann Hood
Dawnson, IL

Dear Drs. Heller:

Your book, *The Carbohydrate Addict's Diet,* was the answer to my prayer and the answer to questions which I had all my life.

I quit smoking and was put on hormones for early menopause 6 years ago. At that time I weighed 128 lbs., which is a good weight for me and one which I worked hard to maintain. In a few months I weighed 147 lbs., was hungry all the time and not pleased with myself. I enrolled in a weight management class which taught me that I must not skip meals (something I had always done before) and that I must eat a high-fiber, low-fat diet and stuff myself with carbohydrates. I managed to lose 12 pounds from that day and until I saw you on the Sally Jessy Raphael Show I gained and lost 5 to 7 pounds enough times to populate an entire country. And no matter what I did I could not get down below 135 lbs. Let me add that I was exercising 5 to 6 hours per week, without exception, 5 hours on my stairclimber and the remainder running on the weekends. So I should have lost weight.

I moaned and carried on to my gynecologist who just told me that hormones make you hungry, and I just had to be careful what I put in my mouth and besides I wasn't fat anyway.

Now I realize that at 5'6" and 135 pounds (which was gradually creeping back up to 141) I wasn't exactly huge but I was very unhappy about my weight. I had called OA to find out where they had meetings in the area, asked God to please help me not lose this battle, and then turned on the TV—and there you were. I have lost 9½ pounds since then, the weight does not fluctuate up and down but goes down and stays there, the diet is easy, one I can live with forever and not feel deprived, and it gets easier and easier as new habits are formed. I no longer crave carbohydrates or feel hungry all the time which is so freeing and empowering for me. I love it. Food has lost its importance due to the Reward Meal concept, which I love. So does my husband, by the way. He has no problem, but just loves getting dessert every night (when dessert was a bad word in our house for years).

This is my story and I can never thank you enough for your work and for writing this marvelous book. . . .

Teddi Forsyth
Bellaire, TX

The fact is, I was "born round" and never understood why. I ate less than my peers, rarely indulged in fat foods, and rarely binged, yet I was always round. The size I wore most of my life was a 12, and often that didn't seem enough. In May 1990, I quit smoking after 30 years because of health problems. I started to gain weight slowly, even though I exercised by walking 3 miles a day and watched my fat intake. Then in March 1991 I was watching television and Cleveland's "Morning Exchange" had Drs. Rachael and Richard Heller talking about their new book. It was as though they were transposed from the television into my living room. Everything they talked about was explaining me. The questions they asked touched my soul and unlocked my special secrets. That day I learned I was a carbohydrate addict. I wrote down the name of the book and the doctors' names, with the intention of going to the bookstore soon. At the same time my mother was in the hospital with terminal cancer, and I didn't think any more about the book.

My mother passed away on April 11, and my family had gathered at my father's home the next day. The same day, a friend of my brother stopped to offer condolences. When I walked into the room, he looked straight at me and said, "God, did you get fat!" I was mortified. No one had ever insulted me like that or hurt me in such a way that I was speechless. After going home crying and feeling despair, I remembered the Drs. Heller and their book.

The next day, I went to the mall and purchased my new bible *(The Carbohydrate Addict's Diet)*. I read it from cover to cover twice and started my new life the next day. That was over one year ago. I lost 35 pounds and I am keeping it off. I have shared this information with many friends and family—I am no longer round.

Thank you Drs. Rachael and Richard Heller for my new life.

Alice Hammond
Orlando, FL

---

Drs. Richard and Rachael Heller are co-directors of The Carbohydrate Addict's Center in New York City.

All correspondence should be addressed to:
Drs. Richard and Rachael Heller
Mt. Sinai School of Medicine—
Box 1194
New York, NY 10029

# Index

# NOTES

# NOTES

# NOTES

# NOTES

# NOTES

# NOTES

# NOTES

# NOTES